A Primer on Stroke

Steven Goins, MD

Neurohospitalist Summit Medical Group

Medical Advisor to Stroke Awareness Oregon

Contents

Introduction and Personal Note	2
ACKNOWLEDGMENTS	3
GLOSSARY	5
Chapter 1. The Brain, Blood Flow and Stroke	20
Chapter 2. TIAs	31
Chapter 3. Recognition of Stroke Symptoms and Need for Immediate Response	38
Chapter 4. Medical Therapies for Acute Stroke	48
Chapter 5. Interventional and Surgical Therapies for Acute Stroke	55
Chapter 6. Secondary Prevention of Stroke	61
Chapter 7. Stroke Outcomes and Overall Impact	70

Introduction and Personal Note

I moved to Bend in 2015 after practicing neurology in the Willamette Valley for 28 years. When I arrived here, I was surprised and disappointed to observe that the use of TPA for treatment of acute stroke was uncommon in Bend. In 2015, only 3% of our patients were receiving TPA, which is well below the national and state averages. When I asked one of our emergency room doctors why our treatment rates were so low, the reply was "because they come in too late". Perhaps there were other reasons, but it eventually became clear that this statement was actually true. Citizens of Central Oregon mostly were not aware how to recognize stroke symptoms, and the victims therefore came in too late to be eligible for treatment. I am extremely happy that this is changing now. Over the following three years, TPA treatment rates soared and an excellent stroke interventional treatment program has been developed at St. Charles Medical Center in Bend. East Cascade EMS is in the process of implementing a regional triage and transport program for stroke patients. More importantly, families are now learning to recognize stroke signs and are beginning to understand that there are effective treatments for this conditions which kills or disables so many of us.

The world is now engaged in a new war against COVID-19. Fighting this new enemy demands our complete attention and all the energy and courage that we possess. However, we cannot overlook the ever-present impact of stroke in our community.

I would like to thank you for choosing to participate in this learning program. A Primer on Stroke was originally conceived as a training program for SAO speakers, but we soon realized that this program would also be helpful for training emergency providers, nurses, doctors and many others who are involved in stroke care. As you read further, it will become apparent how important it is for families and bystanders to recognize symptoms of stroke and to immediately call 911.

The course consists of seven chapters on different topics. Each chapter contains important vocabulary words highlighted in **bold**. All these vocabulary words have also been listed alphabetically in the GLOSSARY. I believe you will find the glossary extremely useful and so it precedes chapter 1. If you skim the glossary, you might feel overwhelmed by the large number of words that are commonly used in communication about stroke. However, if you can read just one chapter at a time and work your way through the 35 pages of text in the chapters, you will become truly well informed about this important topic.

Even though this is a serious subject, we hope that you will find the reading interesting and rewarding. You will certainly learn a lot and become a source of information for your own family and others with whom you work or associate.

Steven Goins, M.D.

ACKNOWLEDGMENTS

Stroke Awareness Oregon is a nonprofit organization based in Central Oregon, dedicated to education of the public and medical community about stroke warning signs and how to access medical care as well as developing resources and support for stroke patients and their families. SAO has made tremendous inroads towards making FAST, a household safety word in Central Oregon. The concept, development and publication of this book has been highly supported by SAO and in particular by Carol Stiles, the Executive Director for Stroke Awareness Oregon.

Viviane Ugalde, MD, specialist in physical medicine and rehabilitation, provided valuable advice and contributed to the writing of Chapter 7.

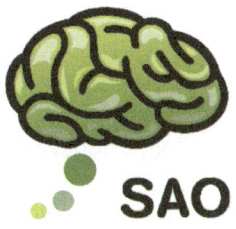

STROKE AWARENESS OREGON

Welcome to **A Primer on Stroke,** written by neurologist Dr. Steve Goins and published by Stroke Awareness Oregon. We believe that knowledge is power, which is why one of our key goals; to educate about stroke causes and prevention and to make F.A.S.T. a household safety word.

Stroke is not the topic one chooses for a social dinner table conversation. In fact, those who experience a stroke often feel ashamed and prefer not to talk about it. But stroke is a critical topic and will strike one in 5 people during their lifetime. If you are in a minority, your risk is one in three. We NEED to have conversations about stroke which is the leading cause of disability worldwide. Every 40 seconds someone in the United States has a stroke and every four minutes, someone dies of a stroke. Eighty percent of strokes are preventable. We want you to know that most strokes are treatable if treatment begins immediately.

We hope you carefully read the seven chapters in this book and learn about the brain, the mechanisms of stroke, stroke treatment options and the absolute necessity to call 9-1-1. Reading five pages a night for a week will make you very knowledgeable about stroke care and will teach you many things of which you were probably unaware. We encourage you to make F.A.S.T. a safety word in your home. F (face drooping A (arm or one sided weakness) S (speech garbled or difficulty speaking) and T (time to call 9-1-1 without hesitation). The information contained in these pages and your rapid response to someone showing signs of a stroke can save the life of someone you love.

If you would like more information about stroke or resources for stroke survivors and their families, please reach out to us. That's what we do!

Carol Stiles

Executive Director

www.strokeawarenessoregon.org 541 323-5641 695 SW Mill View Way, Bend OR 97703

GLOSSARY

ABCs. A mnemonic to remember the assessment of airway, breathing and circulation in an unresponsive person; the initial step before considering cardiopulmonary resuscitation/CPR.

Acute Stroke Ready Hospital. This is the basic designation in the four-tiered classification of stroke centers, recognized by the Joint Commission and American Heart Association.

Agnosia. A neurological term describing how a patient, due to the extent of the brain injury, is unable to process basic sensory information and will be unable to recognize a deficit such as paralysis, blindness or loss of speech.

ASPECTS (Alberta Stroke Program Early CT score). A 10-point semi-quantitative method of using a standard non-contrast brain CT study to evaluate for early ischemic changes: 10 is normal. The scoring system is used to determine whether a patient is eligible for TPA or thrombectomy. Usually, a score of 6 or worse indicates that the ischemic damage has progressed too far and that the risk of hemorrhage is too great to allow treatment with TPA or thrombectomy.

Alteplase. A type of tissue plasminogen activator (TPA) that has been FDA approved for treatment of ischemic stroke.

American Heart Association (AHA). A non-profit organization in the United States that funds cardiovascular and stroke medical research. It is an important clearing house for educational material for the general public related to stroke and heart attack. The AHA also releases important, scientific guideline statements related to stroke treatment.

Aphasia. A disturbance of language function and communication usually related to a brain injury, often involving the left cerebral hemisphere. Aphasia may encompass disorders of language comprehension, reading, speaking and writing in varying degrees.

Apixaban (Eliquis). A relatively new anticoagulant medication, sold under the tradename Eliquis, which functions as a direct inhibitor of factor Xa. It is not dependent on inhibition of vitamin K, unlike warfarin, so it is referred to as a direct acting oral anticoagulant (DOAC).

Apoptosis. A form of programmed cell death; another mechanism for brain cell death after stroke. Unlike neuronal death due to direct trauma, apoptosis occurs gradually through complex biochemical processes.

Arterial dissection. This is the result of a small tear in the inner lining or intima of arteries. The tear leads to the formation of a pouch between the layers of the artery wall that can continue to expand to the point of occluding the artery. The artery dissection can also cause clotting within the artery lumen which can either occlude the artery or embolize to the brain. Dissections can occur in several different arteries but they often involve the carotid arteries or vertebral arteries.

Arteriole. The smallest arteries which terminate on microscopic capillaries.

Arteriolosclerosis. Unlike atherosclerosis which affects larger arteries, arteriolosclerosis causes degeneration of small artery walls. It is related to high blood pressure, diabetes or age. The small artery walls become stiff and lose their normal elasticity in this condition. In the brain, this can lead to either small lacunar strokes or hemorrhages.

Atherosclerosis. A disease of larger arteries caused due to gradual accumulation of cholesterol within the artery walls. The condition begins in adolescence and is common to everyone. Over time, atherosclerosis leads to severe deterioration of the inner lining of the artery and reduces blood flow to the artery but will often lead to clotting or thrombus formation which can embolize. Atherosclerosis is greatly accelerated in individuals with high blood pressure, elevated blood LDL cholesterol, diabetes or who use tobacco.

Atrial fibrillation "A Fib". A common heart arrhythmia which impairs contractions of the upper chambers of the heart or atria. This causes the atria to quiver rather than contract normally. It causes the blood to stagnate and form clots instead of flowing normally into the primary pumping chambers or ventricles of the heart. Eventually, these atrial clots will be ejected by the heart and form emboli capable of causing severe stroke. Atrial fibrillation may be constant, known as chronic atrial fibrillation, or may occur intermittently, known as paroxysmal atrial fibrillation.

Autoregulation. A system within the brain which connects brain nerves to small brain arteries. It highly regulates blood flow into the brain, independent of a person's blood pressure. It can allow blood to continue to flow even when blood pressure is low or it can limit blood flow when blood pressure is too high. When autoregulation is lost due to disease, it can lead to catastrophic effects on brain function.

Basilar artery. A primary artery for the brain which supplies blood flow to the brainstem, cerebellum, thalamus and occipital lobes. It receives blood from the right and left vertebral arteries' inner terminates in the bilateral posterior cerebral arteries which are components of the Circle of Willis.

Body weight support treadmill training. A task-oriented technique for restoring gait after stroke. A person using this technique is supported by a harness suspended from a metal frame which provides support and reduces the weight on the person's feet. This allows higher intensity and more repetitive practice over time compared to conventional therapy.

Brainstem. The posterior part of the brain which forms a continuous part with the spinal cord. It includes the midbrain, pons and medulla oblongata. The brainstem contains centers for control of basic bodily functions including breathing, swallowing, blood pressure control as well as maintaining consciousness. The nuclei of most of the 12 cranial nerves are also located in the brainstem.

Carotid arteries. Paired right and left arteries which supply blood to the anterior 2/3rd of the brain. The common carotid artery exits the chest and enters the neck where it divides to form the external carotid artery, supplying blood to head structures outside of the skull and the internal carotid artery, supplying blood to the eye and the brain.

Carotid endarterectomy. One of the earliest and still commonly performed surgeries to restore blood flow to the brain. It is a treatment for high-grade carotid atherosclerosis with greater than 70% stenosis, which is a major cause of stroke. The procedure involves incising the wall of the carotid artery and removing the diseased inner lining.

Carotid stenting. This is a newer, alternative procedure that is employed instead of carotid endarterectomy. After a catheter is inserted into the groin and then advanced to the level of the carotid artery, a mesh cylinder or stent is expanded into the narrow segment of the carotid artery. This will widen the artery and allow better flow through it while also reducing turbulence of flow. This greatly reduces the likelihood of thrombus formation at the site.

Carotid ultrasound. This is a non-invasive way of assessing flow through the carotid arteries. It uses a computer with an ultrasound transducer. Sound waves passing through the flowing blood produce a signal that can be analyzed. This method only evaluates the carotid artery segment located in the neck and cannot evaluate the carotid artery within the skull or assess major intracranial arteries.

Circle of Willis. The convergence of major arteries, right internal carotid artery, left internal carotid artery and the basilar artery. This joining of the major arteries forms a circle and provides redundancy of blood flow supply to the major cerebral arteries. This is the most important source of collateral blood flow for the brain.

Cerebellum. A major structure of the brain on the brainstem which has connections with the cerebrum and spinal cord. The cerebellum performs the major function of maintaining balance and coordinating limb movements. It also helps in learning new motor skills and has an important function the development of learning, language and personality in children.

Cerebral venous sinus thrombosis. Also known as dural sinus thrombosis or cerebral venous thrombosis, a condition in which a clot forms in the major veins which drain blood away from the brain and back to the heart. This may cause brain or optic nerves to swell and can lead to brain hemorrhages or stroke. The condition could be due to many causes but a disorder of coagulation is the most common cause. Treatment usually requires the use of anticoagulant medications.

Cerebrum. The largest and most complex structure of the human brain, containing extensive cerebral cortex, subcortical white matter and basal ganglia. It is actually divided into two cerebral hemispheres, the right and left hemispheres, which have slightly different functions. In most but not all people, the left hemisphere is referred to as the "dominant" hemisphere because it contains the structures necessary for language. The cerebral hemispheres perform innumerable functions.

CHA2DS2-VASc. A relatively simple scoring system for predicting the risk of thrombus formation and embolism in patients who with atrial fibrillation. Scoring is based on points for congestive heart failure, hypertension, age greater than 75 years, diabetes, prior stroke, peripheral vascular disease and gender. This system is highly important and should be universally used to assess the need for anticoagulation in patients who have experienced atrial fibrillation.

Cholesterol. A complex molecule that is necessary for the formation of cell membranes, certain hormones as well as bile acid for digestion. Cholesterol is produced by the liver but is also obtained from dietary sources, particularly meat. There are multiple forms of cholesterol including LDL cholesterol or low-density lipoprotein cholesterol. LDL cholesterol is also referred to as "bad cholesterol" because it can accumulate within artery walls causing atherosclerosis.

Cilostazol (Pletal). A type of antiplatelet drug sold under the brand name Pletal. It is a relatively weak inhibitor of platelet aggregation. This drug has recently received attention because of its apparent additive effect when combined with either aspirin or clopidogrel for prevention of stroke. A single study of 1201 Japanese patients demonstrated significant reduction of risk of recurrent stroke without an increase in gastrointestinal bleeding.

Cincinnati Stroke Triage Assessment Tool (C-STAT). This is a rapid and easily learned assessment tool for use by emergency responders attending to an individual who may have a stroke. It is being adopted by all emergency response services across Central Oregon as well as the rest of the state to identify patients who may have a large vessel occlusion stroke and who would benefit by direct transport to the closest stroke center capable of performing thrombectomy. C-STAT has only three components to assess: gaze deviation, inability to respond to verbal commands and demonstration of unilateral weakness.

Circle of Willis. The convergence of major arteries, right internal carotid artery, left internal carotid artery and the basilar artery. This joining of the major arteries forms a circle and provides redundancy of blood flow supply to the major cerebral arteries. This is the most important source of collateral blood flow for the brain.

Clopidogrel (Plavix). A type of anti-platelet drug sold under the brand name Plavix. This drug prevents thrombosis by inhibiting the activation of platelets. It does not cause gastric upset unlike aspirin. It is particularly useful in preventing thrombosis after the placement of vascular stents.

Coagulation. A complex process in which liquid blood is converted into a clot or thrombus. This is essential to life to prevent bleeding from minor vascular injuries. Normal coagulation occurs whenever blood components, mainly platelets, are exposed to any breach in the lining of arteries or veins. This will lead to a cascade of chemical processes wherein platelets and fibrin form a firm seal or thrombus over the injured vessel, allowing it to heal. Disorders of coagulation can cause either abnormal bleeding or abnormal, excessive thrombus formation.

Collateral blood flow. If a main artery to the brain becomes occluded, blood may bypass the blockage through accessory arteries that are not ordinarily needed. There are several collateral arteries for the brain, such as those constituting the Circle of Willis, but some individuals may have greater collateral blood flow than others. This can explain why some individuals suffer smaller or no brain injury when major brain arteries become occluded.

Comprehensive Stroke Center. This is the highest designation in the four-tiered classification of stroke centers, recognized by the Joint Commission and American Heart Association. Comprehensive Stroke Centers must possess advanced imaging techniques including MRI, 24-hour neurosurgery and endovascular specialty coverage, 24-hour availability of stroke neurologists and a dedicated neuro ICU.

Constraint induced movement therapy. A form of rehabilitation therapy to enhance arm and hand function affected by brain injury. By restraining the affected arm, it forces the patient to use the impaired upper extremity. The traditional version of the therapy requires the use of a restraining device for 90% of the day but a newer modification involves using the constraint for six hours a day intermittently over 14 days. Although outcomes are improved, the therapy is poorly tolerated by most patients.

Core. The infarct core refers to a portion of the brain that is irrevocably damaged or dead. This is unlike the area of ischemic penumbra which has lost blood supply but is still potentially viable if circulation is restored. If the ratio of penumbra versus core is greater than 1.8 and if the core volume is less than 70 mls, the stroke victim may be a potential candidate for thrombectomy according to the principles of image guided therapy.

Cranial nerves. This refers to the 12 paired nerves that emerge directly from the brain instead of exiting through the spinal cord. These nerves have important special functions for smell, vision, hearing as well as control of eye, facial muscle and throat movement. Injuries to cranial nerves are frequently seen in victims of brainstem strokes.

C-STAT. An acronym for Cincinnati Stroke Triage Assessment Tool, this is a rapid and easily learned assessment tool for use by emergency responders attending to an individual who may have suffered a stroke. It is being adopted by all emergency response services throughout Central Oregon as well as the rest of the state to identify patients who may have suffered a large vessel occlusion stroke and could benefit by direct transport to the closest stroke center, capable of performing thrombectomy. C-STAT has only three components to assess: gaze deviation, inability to respond to verbal commands and demonstration of unilateral weakness.

CT angiogram/CTA. A procedure that requires the use of a computed tomography machine with infusion of contrast material into a vein. This is a rapidly performed procedure commonly in conjunction with a CT scan and sometimes CT perfusion study to evaluate possible stroke and rule out alternative causes for neurological symptoms. It produces highly detailed images of major arteries traveling through the neck and supplying the brain.

CT perfusion/CTP. This test requires the use of a CT screen with infusion of contrast material into a vein. It is usually performed in conjunction with a CTA to evaluate possible stroke. The procedure requires the use of complex software but is considerably faster to and produces similar information as a brain MRI. It can distinguish brain tissue affected by the ischemic penumbra against the core infarct. This is useful for large strokes affecting the cerebral hemispheres but it usually cannot identify small strokes in the brainstem or cerebellum.

CT scan/computerized tomography. A diagnostic imaging test commonly used for brain disorders. It requires the use of computers and rotating x-ray generating machines. The computer will reconstruct multiple two-dimensional images based on the data. This test can be performed very quickly and is a mainstay for evaluating stroke patients. However, ischemic strokes may not be visible on CT scan for several hours which initially limits its usefulness for excluding alternate diagnosis.

Dabigatran (Pradaxa). An anticoagulant medication, sold under the trade name Pradaxa, it functions as a direct inhibitor of factor Xa. It is not dependent on inhibition of vitamin K, unlike warfarin, so it is referred to as a direct acting oral anticoagulant (DOAC).

Dipyridamole. A type of antiplatelet drug sold under the brand name Persantine, this drug prevents thrombosis by inhibiting the activation of platelets but also has vasodilator effects. It does not cause gastric upset like aspirin but may cause headaches. Furthermore, it may have a synergistic effect with aspirin and is often used in combination with it without increasing the gastrointestinal bleeding risk.

Door to groin puncture time. The measurement of time between a stroke patient's arrival in the emergency department until the beginning of the catheterization procedure is the initial step for thrombectomy. This is an important quality measure that is monitored by the Joint Commission for certification of Thrombectomy Capable and comprehensive stroke centers. The goal is to have a door to groin puncture time of less than 90 minutes for at least 50% of all stroke patients.

Door to needle time. The measurement of time between a stroke patient's arrival in the emergency department until the infusion of TPA begins. This is an important quality measure that is monitored by the Joint Commission for Certification of Stroke Centers. The goal is to have a door to needle time of less than 60 minutes for at least 50% of all stroke patients.

Diffusion weighted imaging/DWI. An advanced MRI technique which has now become a routine part of brain MRI studies. It is highly sensitive to certain types of brain changes, particularly brain cell death. In stroke, it can be highly useful in displaying the infarct core. The resolution of DWI is considerably greater than CTP but requires significantly more time to complete the study.

"Drip and ship". An informal but commonly used phrase which means that frontline hospitals can quickly administer TPA to an acute stroke victim and then immediately transport them to a certified stroke center for higher level of care.

Dysphagia. A medical term for swallowing difficulty. There can be many causes of dysphagia but brain injury and stroke are common causes. Dysphagia can be minor and transient, but it can also be severe and may preclude any type of oral nutrition. Patients with dysphagia are at risk for aspirating oral secretions or gastric contents into the lungs. This can cause life-threatening pneumonia. Many patients with severe dysphagia require a nasogastric tube or gastrostomy for nutrition.

Embolic stroke/infarct. Neurological symptoms which persist due to permanent ischemic injury of brain tissue. The mechanism is caused by an embolus which travels from another site and gets lodged into a brain artery.

Embolic TIA (embolic transient ischemic attack). Neurological symptoms which resolve instead of persisting in stroke. It is caused due to an embolus which travels from another site and gets lodged into a brain artery. If the embolus or thrombus lyses or disintegrates, the brain will recover. Patients with embolic TIAs may be at high risk for stroke.

Emergency Medical Service (EMS). Emergency services which respond to illnesses and injuries requiring an urgent response. This may include ground ambulance or air ambulance services. EMS duties include stabilization of victims and then their transportation to hospital for definitive care. EMS can be contacted by dialing 911 which will connect the caller to a trained dispatch operator. EMS providers may have different levels of training and may include paramedics, emergency medical technicians or volunteer firemen.

EMS. An acronym for emergency medical service.

Endocarditis. Inflammation of the heart lining and valves usually due to bacteria but it can also be due to fungi or noninfectious causes. One of the primary dangers of endocarditis is that thrombus can form on the infected heart valves and then can become detached, leading to an embolic stroke.

Enriched environment. Stimulation of the brain by physical and social surroundings. In rehabilitation units, social support, group activities and encouraging self-directed cognitive exercises are found to complement the task-specific training exercises.

Excitotoxic neurotransmitters. This refers to the pathological effect caused by the release of large amounts of excitatory neurotransmitters. Excitatory neurotransmitters such as glutamate or NMDA are molecules used for normal communication between brain cells, but they can lead to brain cell death if released in excessive amounts. This phenomenon of brain cell death occurs in many conditions such as seizures and stroke.

Extended care facility/ECF. An institution devoted to providing medical, nursing or custodial care for disabled individuals over a prolonged period. This often refers to nursing homes which can offer care designed to keep an individual at their current level of functioning but providing fewer rehabilitation services than those offered at skilled nursing facilities. These facilities may be covered by Medicare Part B once Medicare Part A funding has been exhausted. Extended care can also be provided by medical foster homes, assisted living facilities and other types of programs.

FAST. An acronym for Facial drooping, Arm weakness, Speech difficulties and Time to call emergency services, it was originally developed in the United Kingdom to train medical personnel and as an easily memorized method to remember the key ways to recognize and respond to stroke. It has since been adopted worldwide. Training the general public about FAST is one of the primary missions of Stroke Awareness Oregon.

Fibrin. A blood protein that rapidly polymerizes and forms nets, which, along with platelets, entrap red blood cells. These nets will seal wounds involving blood vessels and prevent bleeding. Fibrin is created by the effect of another protein, thrombin, which converts inactive fibrinogen into the highly reactive fibrin protein. Fibrin can also be involved in abnormal clotting that could lead to stroke.

Fibrinogen. This is a chemically inactive precursor blood protein which can be rapidly converted into fibrin, a primary component of naturally occurring and abnormal blood clots.

Fibrinolysis. This is an important chemical process in the blood stream in which the protein plasmin breaks down fibrin nets which are part of clots. The action of fibrinolysis counterbalances the effect of fibrin polymerization so that clotting does not run out of control. Tissue plasminogen activator or TPA acts by producing more plasmin from plasminogen which leads to accelerated fibrinolysis. By activating fibrinolysis, TPA can dissolve clots. This important mechanism is what makes TPA useful in strokes caused by clots or thrombus.

Gastrostomy. A surgically performed opening in the abdominal wall which allows the placement of a gastrostomy tube into the stomach. This allows nutritional formula to be infused directly into the stomach, bypassing the need to swallow food. This is important for stroke patients with dysphagia, the loss of ability to swallow due to brain injury. Gastrostomy may be temporary or permanent. It is often placed as a temporary measure to allow nutrition and prevent life-threatening aspiration pneumonia which can happen if formula enters the lungs.

Get with the Guidelines. An American Heart Association program under which hospitals voluntarily share raw data related to local stroke care and outcomes in order to monitor compliance with American Heart Association stroke care guidelines. St. Charles Medical Center in Bend has been recognized for its performance as a Get with the Guidelines/Stroke Gold Plus with Honor Roll Achievement Award Hospital.

Hemorrhagic conversion. This is a complication occurring in 10% of all strokes and is a feared complication, particularly in bigger strokes. A stroke causing embolus may later lyse or essentially dissolve, allowing blood flow to return into dying arteries in the infarct core. These damaged arteries may rupture, allowing bleeding to occur into already damaged brain tissue. This complication can be life-threatening.

Hemorrhagic stroke. Historically, vascular injuries to the brain are considered either ischemic strokes or hemorrhagic strokes. Hemorrhagic strokes constitute 13% of all strokes. A hemorrhagic stroke occurs when a weakened artery ruptures and bleeds into surrounding brain tissue. Physicians often refer to these as cerebral hemorrhages to avoid confusion surrounding the use of the word stroke. Stroke now commonly refers to ischemic injuries. Hemorrhagic stroke or cerebral hemorrhages may be related to arteriolosclerosis, the same condition that leads to as lacunar strokes, but they can also be caused by blood vessel malformations, aneurysms or tumors.

Heparin. A naturally occurring protein used intravenously in concentrated forms, it works as a powerful anticoagulant. It inhibits the formation of thrombin and thereby inhibits the formation of clots and prevents the growth of the clot, allowing natural occurring fibrinolysis to dissolve the thrombus. Heparin is used for several medical problems including myocardial infarction and deep vein thrombosis. It has returned as an important treatment for stroke to tackle clots that do not completely occlude an artery. Due to its extremely short action duration, it can be infused intravenously at a constant rate for close monitoring. Newer drugs which have been modified from heparin include enoxaparin. These newer drugs have longer duration of action and are easier to use in certain situations.

Herniation. The brain is constrained within the rigid skull. If brain swelling occurs from an injury such as ischemic stroke or hemorrhage, it may lead the brain to shift across structures inside the skull leading to the compression of other brain structures. It can also cause the compression of arteries which can result in ischemia or additional strokes. This can be a spiraling cascade that ultimately leads to death. An enlarged pupil in an unresponsive patient is a warning sign for one type of herniation. Herniation is an emergency that may require treatment with medications that dehydrate the brain or may require brain surgery.

Holter monitor. A machine that records a heart rhythm for over 24 to 48 hours. The device is contained in a small battery-powered box which connects to electrodes placed over the chest. It is useful for screening for paroxysmal atrial fibrillation. Newer monitoring systems such as Ziopatch or loop recorders offer the advantage of recording for longer durations and are thus replacing Holter monitors.

Internal carotid arteries. Paired right and left arteries which supply blood to the anterior 2/3rd of the brain. The common carotid artery exits the chest and enters the neck where it divides to form the external carotid artery, supplying blood to head structures outside of the skull and the internal carotid artery, supplying the eye and the brain. The two internal carotid arteries terminate on the Circle of Willis. Atherosclerosis buildup at the origin of the internal carotid artery is a major cause of stroke.

Ischemia/Ischemic. A medical term meaning inadequate blood supply to body tissue, ischemia of brain tissue is the primary mechanism of brain injury in stroke.

Ischemic stroke/infarct. The type of stroke resulting from the blockage of blood supply to the brain, it causes 87% of all strokes if hemorrhagic strokes are included. In most discussions, the word stroke implies ischemic stroke and hemorrhagic stroke is considered separately as cerebral hemorrhage.

Image-based therapy. A concept developed in the last decade which employs data from advanced imaging techniques such as MRI or CT perfusion to assess the viability and extent of the ischemic penumbra to make decisions about attempting the reperfusion of brain tissue by thrombectomy and possibly TPA in selected cases. This is in contrast to time-based therapy which considers the duration of symptoms to estimate brain tissue viability.

Lacunar stroke/infarct. These are small ischemic strokes that usually occur in the distribution of small arteries branching off from larger arteries at the base of the brain. Lacunar strokes may not cause any symptoms but can lead to severe paralysis if the stroke occurs in a vital structure of the brain. The small arteries collapse and thrombose as a result of arteriolosclerosis caused due to high blood pressure, diabetes, age or occasional genetic causes.

Lacunar TIA. A transient neurological event that precedes a lacunar stroke. Lacunar stroke symptoms often stutter for reasons that are yet unclear.

Large vessel disease. An informal medical term that refers to diseases, particularly atherosclerosis but also dissection and other less common diseases, that affect large arteries in contrast to the different set of diseases that affect small arteries or arterioles.

Last seen normal. This refers to the time between when a stroke victim was last seen without symptoms till the time of their arrival in the emergency department. This time must be less than 4.5 hours for a person to be considered for treatment with TPA, after which the risk of hemorrhage becomes too great. If a patient wakes up with stroke symptoms, the last seen normal time may be when the person went to bed. In the past, last seen normal greater than 6 hours was considered disqualification for thrombectomy, but this is now being replaced by image-guided therapy protocols.

LDL cholesterol/Low density lipoprotein cholesterol. Cholesterol is an important complex molecule necessary for the body. However, not all cholesterol is good. LDL cholesterol, referred to as "bad cholesterol", is a specific type of cholesterol which accumulates in artery walls leading to atherosclerosis. LDL cholesterol is produced in the liver but a substantial component is supplemented from our diet.

Low-flow TIA. A less common type of TIA caused by a sudden drop in blood pressure in a person with critical narrowing or stenosis of a brain artery. It is not caused by an embolus, therefore treatment needs to address the cause of blood pressure fluctuations and possibly requires the treatment of the blockage. Anti-platelet drugs may be prescribed but cannot correct the underlying problem.

Lipohyalinosis. An older term describing arteriolosclerosis changes in the small arteries of the brain. This condition is not completely understood but is caused by high blood pressure, diabetes, age, genetics and inflammation. These changes are associated with increased risk for lacunar strokes, cerebral hemorrhages and certain forms of dementia.

LVO stroke/Large vessel occlusion stroke. Strokes caused by embolic occlusion of major brain arteries including the internal carotid artery, middle cerebral artery and basilar artery. These comprise over a third of all strokes and are significantly more likely to lead to devastating neurological handicap or death. Since these sudden occlusions are usually due to larger emboli or thrombus, TPA is less likely to be effective. Urgent thrombectomy has revolutionized care for many of these previously catastrophic strokes.

LVO/wake-up stroke triage protocol. Triage is a general medical term which implies determining the priority of treatment based on a patient's condition. LVO stroke victims require rapid triage and transport to the nearest hospital capable of thrombectomy even if it means bypassing a nearby hospital. The East Cascade Emergency Medical Services Council, constituted by representatives from every fire and EMS agency within the greater Central Oregon Region, has approved and is in the process of adopting a triage protocol to ensure rapid transport of LVO stroke victims to the closest hospital with thrombectomy capability. This usually involves transport by ground or air ambulance to Charles Medical Center in Bend.

Migraine aura. This is a remarkably common and usually benign occurrence, affecting millions of people each year, in which brain function is altered or suppressed by an electrical wave spreading slowly across the brain cortex. This is usually a transient disturbance of vision involving an expanding C-shaped zig-zag pattern which may be followed by a headache. But the aura may affect other brain functions including speech or motor control, resembling a stroke. Migraine aura is one of the most common stroke mimics. Indications of an aura include gradual onset, association with headache and a tendency for lifetime recurrence.

MRI/magnetic resonance imaging. An advanced imaging technique which revolutionized the diagnosis of many neurological diseases. The test involves computer generated images of the brain obtained from recording radio waves bouncing off brain tissue water molecules aligned or synchronized in a strong magnetic field. Unlike X-rays or CT scans, the test does not involve ionizing radiation. Variations or different MRI sequences allow looking at the brain in different ways. Diffusion restriction MRI (DWI) is a highly sensitive method of identifying acute strokes in the acute period. This can be extremely helpful to physicians in locating the vascular distribution and cause of a stroke.

Multi-infarct dementia. A type of vascular dementia, this is the second most common cause of dementia following Alzheimer's and is possibly a preventable form of dementia. It often occurs due to chronic smoldering small vessel disease or from multiple small strokes or a major stroke.

Nasogastric tube/NG tube. A plastic tube which is inserted through a nasal passage into the esophagus and finally into the stomach. It is a temporary measure employed to provide fluids and nutrition to a patient who is unable to swallow safely.

Neuroprotective drugs. Drugs which are designed to prevent neuron cell death due to chemical processes that occur after the initial ischemic insult. These drugs aim to slow oxidative stress, mitochondrial dysfunction, excitotoxicity and multiple other processes that contribute to brain cell death in stroke. Currently, despite intensive and encouraging research, there are no neuroprotective drugs which have proven to improve the outcome with regard to stroke.

No reflow phenomena. The failure of blood to be restored to ischemic brain tissue after the physical obstruction has been removed. This is probably due to the irreversible ischemic damage caused to small blood vessels.

Neglect. An informal term used to describe the many complex forms of agnosia in which due to the extent of the brain injury, the stroke victim is unable to process basic sensory information and recognize a deficit such as paralysis, blindness or loss of speech. A stroke patient may ignore everything in the room on the side of their paralysis or may or not even recognize their arm as belonging to them.

Penumbra. The infarct penumbra is the portion of the brain that has lost blood supply but has not yet died and can possibly survive if circulation is restored. This is in contrast to the core which suffers irreversible damage. If the ratio of penumbra versus core is greater than 1.8 and if the core volume is less than 70 mls, the stroke victim may be a potential candidate for thrombectomy according to the principles of image guided therapy.

Permissive hypertension. A component of treatments for acute stroke, blood pressure initially may be greatly elevated in stroke patients, presumably as a biological reflex attempting to restore blood flow to ischemic brain tissue via collateral circulation. Permissive hypertension is a medical decision to allow blood pressure to rise up to 220/110 for 24 hours or possibly longer to enhance this effect.

PFO/Patent foramen ovale. The foramen ovale is an opening between the two atria or upper chambers of the heart and is required to allow oxygen carrying blood from the mother's placenta to the heart of the fetus. The hole, or foramen, is supposed to close at birth but remains partially open in up to 1 in 4 people. This persistence of the foramen ovale is called a patent foramen ovale or PFO. PFO rarely causes symptoms in most people but it can become a conduit for venous clots to cross into the arteries and travel to the brain.

Plasmin. An important blood protein that degrades fibrin clots, by a process known as fibrinolysis. Without the effect of plasmin, blood would be constantly clotting in an uncontrollable manner. Plasmin is only present when it is carefully released from an inactive form, fibrinogen, through complex biological systems. However, TPA, is a pharmacological agent which can convert plasminogen into plasmin to dissolve clots.

Plasminogen. An important blood protein which is always present in blood but remains inactive until it is converted into plasmin.

Plasticity. An incredible property of the brain by which many brain functions can be shifted from one location to another and even to the opposite side of the brain. This property is most fully developed in childhood and is a fundamental component of learning; however, plasticity is present throughout life and is a basis for recovery after stroke. Rehabilitation significantly enhances brain plasticity after injury.

Platelets. Also called thrombocytes, platelets are tiny, abundant blood cells which adhere and clump at sites of blood vessel injury. Platelet clumping combines with fibrin polymerization to form thrombus or clots. This is necessary for life although abnormal thrombus formation causes disease and is a major factor in stroke.

POLST/Provider Orders for Life-Sustaining Treatment. A standardized, legally recognized document which clarifies a person's decisions regarding life sustaining therapies including CPR and tube feedings. POLST is usually indicated for medically fragile people or those with shortened life expectancy. POLST forms originated in Oregon in 1991 but are recognized in 42 states now.

Post-stroke cognitive impairment/dementia. An important and potentially preventable cause of dementia which is secondary only to Alzheimer's disease. It may occur after a single stroke or after multiple strokes or as a consequence of chronic brain tissue ischemia due to chronic small vessel disease.

Primary Stroke Center. An intermediate designation in the four-tiered classification of stroke centers recognized by the Joint Commission and American Heart Association, Comprehensive Stroke Centers. Primary Stroke Centers must have a dedicated stroke program; they are further required to collect extensive data to monitor performance and adherence to standards of care.

Primary stroke prevention. A strategy or goal applicable to all patients who have never had a stroke. The aim is to correct and improve lifestyle and health factors which have shown to greatly increase the risk of stroke over a lifetime. These factors include high blood pressure, diabetes, elevated LDL cholesterol and tobacco use, in addition to atrial fibrillation, sleep apnea, obesity and other health conditions.

Physical medicine and rehabilitation specialist/Physiatrist. Medical doctors who have completed training in the specialty of Physical Medicine and Rehabilitation and may be subspecialty certified in Brain Injury Medicine, Hospice and Palliative Medicine, Neuromuscular Medicine, Pain Medicine, Pediatric Rehabilitation Medicine, Spinal Cord Injury Medicine and/or Sports Medicine.

Paroxysmal atrial fibrillation/Paroxysmal "a-fib". An intermittent variation of atrial fibrillation which impairs contractions of the upper chambers of the heart or atria. This causes the atria to quiver rather than contract normally, leading blood to stagnate and form clots rather than flowing normally into the main pumping chambers or ventricles of the heart. Eventually, these atrial clots will be ejected by the heart and form emboli capable of causing severe stroke. Since treatment requires the use of anticoagulant medications, accurate detection of paroxysmal a-fib is extremely important. It is a challenge that is now being addressed by newer long-term detection heart monitoring systems.

Rivaroxaban (Xarelto). A relatively new anticoagulant medication, sold under the trade name Xarelto, which functions as a direct inhibitor of factor Xa. It is not dependent on the inhibition of vitamin K, unlike warfarin, so it is referred to as a direct acting oral anticoagulant (DOAC).

Secondary stroke prevention. The strategy applied to stroke survivors, who, in general, have a 4-fold increased risk of future strokes. This includes extensive diagnostic studies and management of stroke risk factors including hypertension, elevated LDL cholesterol, diabetes, tobacco use, atrial fibrillation and vascular stenosis. Treatment with antithrombotic medication and lipid lowering drugs are standard procedure. Some patients will benefit from procedures to correct vascular stenosis.

Skilled nursing facility/SNF. A facility offering a complex level of care, including registered nurses, physical therapists, speech therapists and occupational therapists. After hospital discharge, stroke survivors may stay at a SNF as a transitional step before returning home. Ordinarily, SNF are not intended as long-term care facilities. Medicare Part A will pay only for up to 100 days for admission to a SNF.

Small vessel disease. An informal medical term referring to diseases which affect small arteries or arterioles. This commonly refers to arteriolosclerosis caused by high blood pressure, diabetes, age or genetic causes rather than the cholesterol deposition seen in large vessel disease.

Small vessel TIA. See also lacunar TIA. A transient neurological event that precedes a lacunar stroke. Lacunar stroke symptoms often stutter due to reasons that are unclear.

Small vessel stroke. Synonymous to lacunar stroke, these are small ischemic strokes that usually occur in the distribution of small arteries branching out from larger arteries at the base of the brain. Lacunar strokes may not cause any symptoms but are capable of causing severe paralysis if the stroke occurs in a vital structure of the brain. The small arteries collapse and thrombose causing arteriolosclerosis due to high blood pressure, diabetes, age or at times genetic causes. These strokes may contribute to vascular dementia.

Stenosis. A medical term that implies narrowing of a structure. Stenosis of an artery, such as carotid stenosis, may lead to reduced blood flow but can also cause turbulence of flow and increase the risk of a thrombus or embolus formation.

Stent retriever. A type of device used for thrombectomy in which a delicate wire net is passed around a thrombus and is then contracted, capturing the thrombus for removal, thus known as clot retrieval. Other retrieval methods include direct aspiration or use of corkscrew devices.

Stroke mimics. Conditions which may have symptoms that resemble ischemic stroke. These may include migraine with aura, Todd's paralysis after an epileptic seizure, psychological conditions such as conversion disorders and multiple other brain disorders. Distinguishing between ischemic stroke and stroke mimics is a significant challenge for ED physicians and neurologists who are considering treatment with TPA. Up to 1 in 20 patients presenting with paralysis may ultimately prove to have a stroke mimic.

STROKE ONE. A code word used by the St. Charles Medical System and referring EMS systems in Central Oregon to alert all members of the stroke care team about the arrival of a stroke victim. This activates a STROKE ONE care pathway and facilitates rapid coordination among the multiple members of a stroke care team. In other areas, the term Stroke Alert is often used as the code word.

Task-specific training. A strategy for rehabilitation used for stroke survivors. Rather than requiring exercises focused on correcting deficits such as muscular weakness, the patient is directed to repeatedly perform actions that are useful for life, such as reaching for a cup or pouring liquid.

Telemetry. Remote monitoring of the heart rhythm by a telemetry nurse. This is performed on hospitalized stroke patients to look for possible paroxysmal atrial fibrillation.

Tenecteplase/TNK. Another type of tissue plasminogen activator which offers advantages over alteplase and may become the preferred thrombolytic drug in the near future. It is marketed under the trade name TNKase and is commonly referred to as TNK. Tenecteplase is less expensive than alteplase, but more importantly, it can be infused rapidly rather than infused over an hour as required for alteplase. This may allow improved effectiveness and is a less complicated alternative when the stroke victim is about to be transported from a smaller hospital to a stroke center.

Therapeutic hypothermia. A neuroprotective therapy designed to slow oxidative stress, mitochondrial dysfunction, excitotoxicity and multiple other processes that contribute to brain cell death after brain ischemia. Hypothermia is now standard care for patients who have suffered cardiac arrest or for newborns with birth asphyxia. Hypothermia has not found a treatment role in stroke probably due to practical problems in cooling of conscious patients.

Thrombectomy. A procedure performed by a physician, typically a neurosurgeon, interventional radiologist or stroke neurologist, working with an interventional team. The interventionalist inserts a catheter into a peripheral artery and passes the catheter tip up through the aorta until it reaches the occluded cerebral artery. Then, the clot can be captured and pulled out; this is known as clot retrieval. Thrombectomy can traditionally be performed within 6 hours after symptom onset but can also be done beyond this window, up to 24 hours, if imaging studies show viable tissue or penumbra in the ischemic area.

Thrombectomy Capable Stroke Center. This is a new and second highest designation in the four-tiered classification of stroke centers, recognized by the Joint Commission and American Heart Association. These hospitals meet requirements of Primary Stroke Centers and also provide 24/7 coverage by stroke interventional specialists with documented experience of performing thrombectomy for stroke.

TIA. Acronym for transient ischemic attack. Although it is sometimes referred to as a "mini-stroke", it is caused due to a reversible malfunction of brain tissue because of a temporary blockage of blood flow to a part of the brain or eye. Usually the warning lasts only a few minutes and might be ignored by the victim. It is a signal that something is wrong and it may lead to a stroke. This is an opportunity to remember FAST.

Time-based therapy. A concept that involves using the duration of symptoms' time interval to estimate brain tissue viability. Treatment of acute stroke with TPA can be allowed for up to 3 hours after the onset of symptoms according to the FDA. Later studies have demonstrated that TPA can be used for up to 4.5 hours although its greatest effectiveness has been seen in patients who have been treated early. The high risk of hemorrhage precludes using TPA beyond 4.5 hours.

Todd's paralysis. Temporary brain malfunction occurring after an epileptic seizure. This may be paralysis or aphasia or other neurological symptoms. Todd's paralysis usually resolves within minutes or hours but can be mistaken for a stroke.

TPA/Tissue plasminogen activator. Although the term actually refers to a group of similar drugs, it is commonly used as another name for alteplase, a specific type of TPA. Alteplase is marketed under the trade name Activase. It is currently the only tissue plasminogen activator that has been FDA approved for the treatment of ischemic stroke.

Transcarotid artery revascularization/TCAR. A new advanced stent treatment for carotid stenosis. After a catheter is inserted directly into the carotid artery, a system is introduced to temporarily reverse blood flow in the internal carotid artery before a mesh cylinder or stent is expanded into the narrow segment of the carotid artery. This prevents debris from flowing to the brain and increases the safety of the procedure. The stent widens the artery and allows better flow through it while also reducing the turbulence of flow. This greatly reduces the likelihood of thrombus formation at the site.

Transient ischemic attack. Also known as "TIA". Although it is sometimes referred to as a "mini-stroke", it is caused by reversible malfunction of brain tissue due to a temporary blockage of blood flow to a part of the brain or eye. Usually the warning lasts for only a few minutes and might be ignored by the victim. This is a signal that something is wrong and can lead to a stroke. This is the time to remember FAST.

Transient global amnesia. A relatively uncommon neurological disorder of unknown cause in which a person abruptly loses all capacity to remember any new information for more than a minute or less.

These people are incapacitated by confusion and fear for hours but typically achieve complete recovery by the following day. The condition affects older people and may occasionally entail recurrence. The condition may resemble a stroke because of the sudden onset, but it is a benign condition which has no connection to stroke or stroke-related risk factors.

Vascular dementia. Sometimes known as multi-infarct dementia and Binswanger disease, this is the second most common cause of dementia following Alzheimer's disease and is a preventable form of dementia. It often occurs due to chronic smoldering small vessel disease or multiple small strokes or a major stroke.

Vertebral arteries. Paired major arteries in the neck which converge into the basilar artery and supply the majority of blood flow to the posterior 1/3rd of the brain. Often, one of the vertebral arteries are dominant. Unlike the internal carotid arteries, the vertebral arteries receive collateral flow. The location of the vertebral arteries renders them susceptible to dissection.

Vertigo. An unpleasant sensation of motion while a person is still, often accompanied by nausea and impaired balance. While vertigo is usually related to inner ear disturbances, it can also happen with strokes involving the brainstem. Vertigo from brainstem strokes is usually combined with other neurological symptoms such as double vision or numbness or weakness. MRI may or may not demonstrate the stroke if performed too early. Evaluation of vertigo is a common challenge for emergency room doctors.

Wake-up stroke. The situation when a patient wakes up with stroke symptoms that were not present before they fell asleep. Previously, the last seen normal time needed to be, without doubt, less than 4.5 hours for a person to be eligible for treatment with TPA. Now, image-guided therapy, using CT perfusion and MRI, allows treatment for many patients who suffer wake-up strokes.

Warfarin (Coumadin). An older, inexpensive but extremely important and highly effective anticoagulant medication marketed under the trade name Coumadin. Warfarin inhibits thrombus formation by blocking the effect of vitamin K which is vital for the formation of proteins needed for clot formation. The effect takes several days to transpire and requires precision monitoring of laboratory tests (prothrombin time or INR). The World Health Organization lists warfarin as one of the safest and most effective medications necessary in the health system.

Ziopatch. The tradename for a relatively new cardiac rhythm monitoring device which is currently used for the detection of paroxysmal atrial fibrillation. It is capable of continuously monitoring heart rhythms for 24 hours daily for up to 14 days which allows considerably improved detection compared to holter monitoring. Moreover, it is extremely convenient for the patient since it involves wearing only a small adhesive patch containing an electronic sensor. Disadvantages include the cost and the long-time interval preceding the final results. Ziopatch is likely to be followed by similar and increasingly more convenient systems including the Apple Watch.

Chapter 1. The Brain, Blood Flow and Stroke

Even in ancient times, people recognized symptoms of stroke as sudden collapse followed by death or paralysis. Hippocrates described symptoms of stroke over 2,400 years ago. In the second century A.D., Galen coined the term apoplexy, a Greek word meaning "struck down in violence". The word apoplexy was used in various ways to describe stroke symptoms well into the 20th century. Now, the word **stroke** is more commonly used. However, this is imprecise as it refers to several types of brain injuries. This includes ischemic stroke related to loss of blood supply to the brain. Hemorrhagic stroke, which means bleeding in the brain tissue, is often related to some of the underlying diseases that cause ischemic stroke. Furthermore, there are less commonly encountered brain injuries such as venous infarct stroke or even metabolic strokes caused due to chemical changes in the brain cell metabolism, which outstrip the energy supply. Usually, when the word stroke is used, it means ischemic stroke, which is the most common type of stroke. In ischemic stroke, the loss of blood circulation to the brain leads to tissue damage and subsequent disability. This primer will focus on ischemic stroke, referred to as "stroke" hereafter. Ischemic stroke constitutes 87% of all types of strokes.

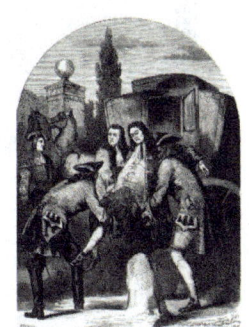

'Hippocrates, engraving by Peter Paul Rubens, 1638.' Public domain.

'King George attacked by a fit of apoplexy'. Public domain

The British physician William Harvey first described and recognized blood circulation in the 1600s. It was not until the 1800s that arterial blockage began to be recognized as a cause for stroke. Today, we know that there are multiple types of strokes and many different causes for each type. Regardless of the cause, the consequence of a stroke primarily depends on the part of the brain injured and the degree of the injury.

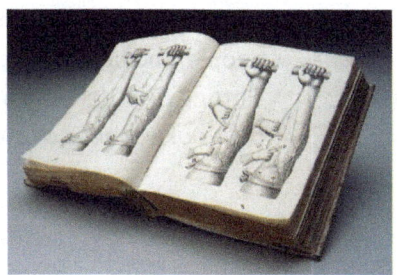

'De Motu Cordis' by William Harvey. Wellcome Library. CC-BY4.0.

A basic breakdown of stroke causes includes three general categories:

- **Large vessel disease**, in particular due to atherosclerosis, the result of cholesterol accumulation within the artery wall with subsequent deterioration and eventual **thrombosis** (clot formation). However, multiple other diseases can also damage large vessels.

- Small vessel disease, mostly referred to as **lacunar infarcts**. These are small strokes caused by the degeneration of small penetrating brain arteries or

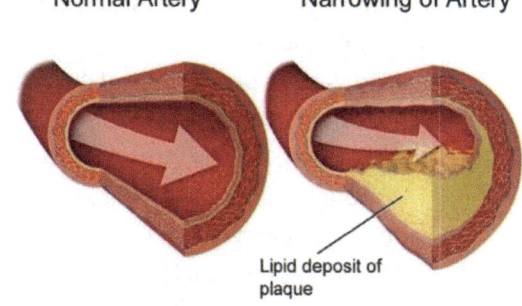

'Atherosclerosis'. Oregon State University. CC-BY-SA-2.0.

arteriolosclerosis, leading to the occlusion of the arteries. The primary causes are age, high blood pressure and diabetes. The kidneys and eyes are other organs affected by arteriolosclerosis. Though less commonly, atherosclerosis from cholesterol build up can also cause lacunar infarcts.

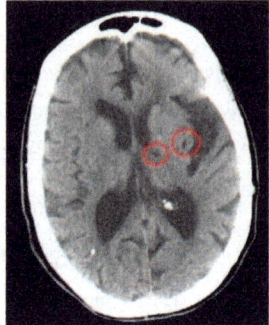

'Lacunar strokes'.
Mikael Haggstrom. CC-BY-SA-3.0.

- **Embolic strokes**. These strokes are caused by an embolus, which are clots or debris that originate elsewhere in the body and travel up to the brain arteries and occlude a vital artery. An embolus can form in the heart or an area of atherosclerosis or even travel from other sites in the body. One of the most common causes of cardiac emboli is atrial fibrillation. Patent foramen ovale, difficult to diagnose, is another relatively common cause of stroke across all ages, even in newborns. The patent foramen ovale is a persistent hole between the right atrium and left atrium of the heart. This hole is necessary for life in the womb but is supposed to close at birth. However, in one out of four healthy people, the patent foramen ovale remains open. Blood clotting disorders are a less common but perhaps overlooked cause or contributor to embolic strokes.

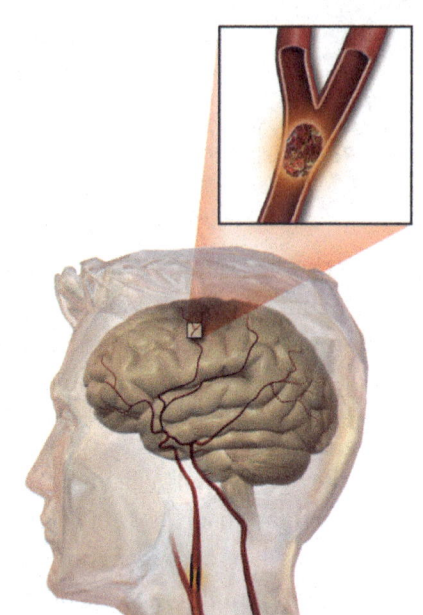

'Embolic stroke'. Blaussen Medical Communications, Inc. CC-BY-3.0.

Why is knowledge about strokes so important? Stroke is the fifth most common cause of death in the United States.

- It is the greatest cause of disability in the United States.
- The social and economic burden of stroke on individuals, families and their communities is tremendous.
- Strokes are preventable. Lifestyle choices beginning in adolescence greatly impact the occurrence of stroke throughout one's lifetime. Strokes in teenagers or young adults are particularly tragic. Attempts to reduce the incidence of stroke in a community or individuals through education, dietary changes, blood pressure control and tobacco cessation is known as **primary prevention**. In the past, primary prevention was believed to be the responsibility of health professionals, but in truth, it is everyone's responsibility, particularly parents, grandparents and community leaders. Stroke Awareness Oregon (SAO) is a community organization focused on the primary prevention of stroke.

- In general, strokes are treatable. Previously, strokes that could cause permanent disability or were fatal can now mostly be treated with **thrombolytic drugs** such as **TPA** or **thrombectomy**, also referred to as **clot retrieval**. The success of treatment depends on the availability of knowledgeable physicians and highly trained and coordinated stroke teams. Since the brain is highly dependent on a continuous blood supply, brain injury occurs very rapidly in stroke and completely successful treatment must be provided within a short span of time, usually requiring minutes but occasionally lasting for a few hours. Since individuals who have suffered a stroke usually are unaware of the fact, it is essential that their companions or bystanders recognize the symptoms of stroke and call 911 immediately to ensure there is a chance for successful treatment. Giving everyone in a community training to be familiar with **FAST** (face, arm, speech and time) is extremely important, but up till now, there have been no nationally organized efforts to education the entire population about FAST. SAO is a grassroots organization consisting of concerned Oregon citizens who hope to make a difference.
- Individuals who have suffered a stroke or **transient ischemic attack (TIA)** are at high risk for further strokes and disability. In order to prevent premature death and disability for this group, the medical profession follows complex guidelines for an extensive medical evaluation and treatment. This is called **secondary prevention**. The **American Heart Association** provides extensive and frequently updated guidelines for health professionals treating acute symptoms stroke responsible for secondary prevention. These updated guidelines are published regularly and are based on extensive scientific research and the opinions of recognized medical experts.

For Americans, lifetime stroke risk is 25%. Essentially, this means that one in every four people that you know, including members of your close family, will suffer a stroke in their lifetime. For patients who have experienced one stroke, there is a roughly 30% of recurrence within the next five years. A total of 795,000 new cases of strokes happen in the United States annually. Two-thirds of stroke survivors are disabled as a result of stroke.

The Brain

The most important organ of our body controls all bodily functions, processes information from all the senses, stores all memories and is the seat of consciousness. The brain contains 100 billion cells and each cell or neuron shares physical connections with tens of thousands of other brain cells. In fact, most of the brain's substance is composed of connections or synapses between the many neurons. For the purpose of understanding the impact of stroke, one needs to know a few things about the different parts of the brain. We can divide the brain into three basic parts, the cerebrum, cerebellum and the brainstem.

- The **brainstem** comprises several components and forms the connection between the cerebrum and spinal cord. All of our life control centers, for breathing, regulation of blood pressure and heart rate as well as our brain system for keeping us awake or asleep are located in the brainstem. Additionally, the brainstem is where the centers or nuclei for the 12 **cranial nerves** are located. These cranial nerves are involved in smell, vision, control of eye movements, hearing, vocal cord movement and swallowing. Even small strokes in the brainstem can create serious handicaps due to injuries in the cranial nerve nuclei and because extremely important pathways between the cerebrum and spinal cord pass through the brainstem. Brainstem strokes are often caused due to the occlusion of small blood vessels: these small arterial occlusions can lead to severe handicaps or death.

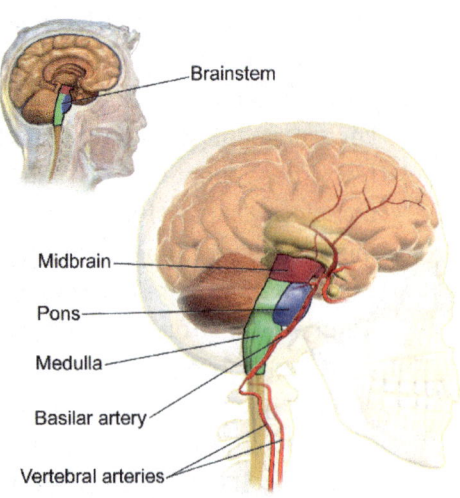

'The brainstem receives blood via the vertebral arteries'. Medical gallery of Blausen Medical 2014. CC-BY-3.0.

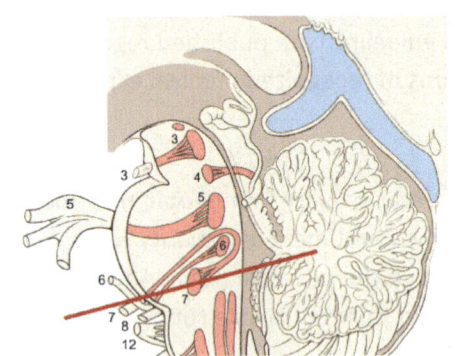

'Cross section of the brainstem showing multiple nuclei of the 10 pair of cranial nerves that emerge from it'. Patrick J Lynch, medical illustrator. CC-BY-2.5

- The **cerebellum** is the part of the brain closely involved in balance and coordination. It is also believed to have an important role in learning in childhood. Remarkably, patients who suffer strokes limited to the cerebellum can often recover with only moderate handicaps. Strokes in the cerebellum, similar to strokes elsewhere in the brain, can lead to swelling during the first week. Since the cerebellum is encased by the skull and membranes, it can cause fatal compression of the brainstem as it swells.

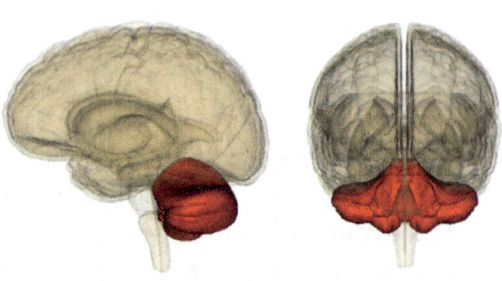

'Cerebellum'. Images are generated by Life Science Databases (LSDB). CC-BY-SA-2.1jp.

- The **cerebrum** consists of two separate hemispheres, the right and the left hemispheres. The motor output for each hemisphere crosses in the brainstem. Likewise, sensory input from our limbs crosses to the opposite side in the cerebrum. The effect is that injury to one hemisphere leads to motor and sensory problems in the opposite side of the body. Furthermore, visual input from our eyes also crosses in a complex way, thus injury to one hemisphere can lead to a loss of visual perception on the opposite side. The cerebral hemispheres are the primary computers of our brain. This is where the mind processes all the information from the outside world and forms speech and ideas. The left hemisphere is commonly referred to as the dominant hemisphere because it is where the language centers reside in 92% of people. It is the hemisphere that controls one's right hand, if one is right-handed. Left-handed people use the right hemisphere for motor control but can use either the right or left hemisphere or both for language. Many different types of strokes can affect cerebral hemispheres. Emboli coming from the heart or from atherosclerotic large arteries can travel from the main arteries to different parts of the cerebral hemispheres. Small strokes can be related to degeneration of small penetrating arteries. We often refer to these small strokes as lacunar infarcts. Lacunar is derived from Latin meaning small pit. Some individuals can suffer multiple lacunar strokes and not show any symptoms, but if a lacunar stroke occurs in a vital area, severe paralysis can occur.

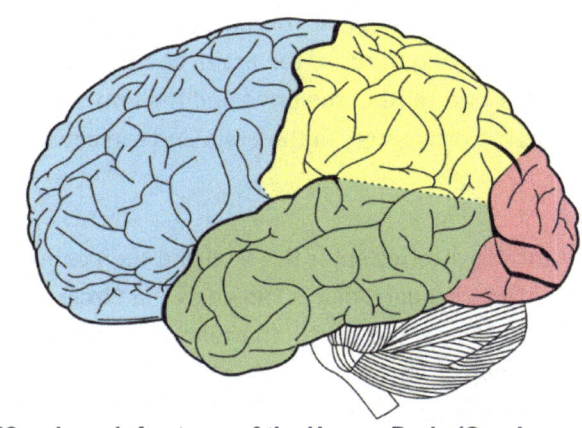

'Cerebrum'. Anatomy of the Human Body (Gray's Anatomy). Public domain.

Blood Circulation to the Brain

The brain and, to a lesser extent, the kidneys have a very high requirement for blood flow and oxygen in comparison to all other tissues in the body. A total of 15% of the body's cardiac output goes to the brain, supplying oxygen and glucose and returning carbon dioxide, lactic acid and other waste products back to the body. Without constant oxygen delivery, brain cells can die within minutes. Incomplete cardiac arrest, irreversible brain damage begins within eight minutes. When a major artery to the brain is occluded, nearly 2 million brain cells die every minute due to a lack of blood flow. Glucose is essentially the only energy source that can be used by brain cells, although in certain situations the brain can survive on ketones, which is a product of fat metabolism.

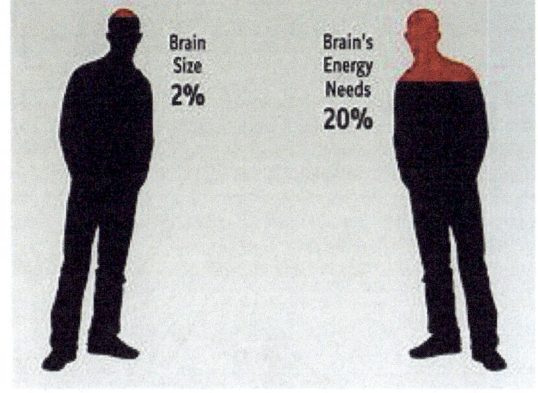

'Brain weight versus energy requirements'. ...edu

Delivery of blood and nutrients to the brain is dependent on several factors.

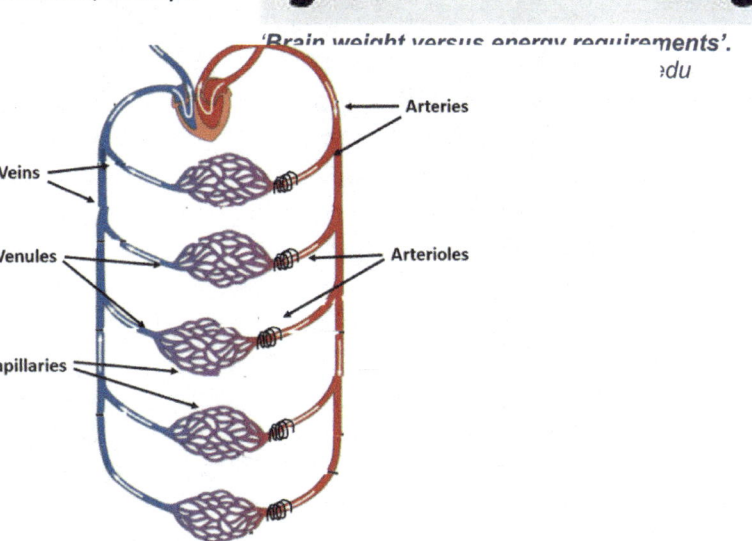

As blood is pumped out of the heart through the aorta, it is channeled through four major arteries before it enters the skull. This includes the right and left **internal carotid arteries** which supply blood to the anterior two thirds of the brain, and the right and left vertebral arteries which supply blood to the posterior one-third of the brain and the important brainstem structures. Clots or emboli can travel from the heart to any artery in the brain and can cause multiple strokes involving multiple artery territories.

The carotid arteries enter the skull and then connect with each other through what is known as the **Circle of Willis**. The Circle of Willis is the most important of several collateral blood flow systems in the human body.

'Circulation diagram labeling the Diffe Alan Sved. CC-BY-SA-4.0.

Collateral blood flow can protect the brain if a major artery becomes occluded. However, significantly, 40% patients who experience a complete occlusion of one of their carotid arteries can be without any symptoms due to good collateral blood flow, primarily by the Circle of Willis. Unfortunately, sudden complete occlusion of a carotid artery will commonly lead to a devastating stroke involving most of the cerebral hemisphere with complete paralysis of one side along with multiple other neurological handicaps.

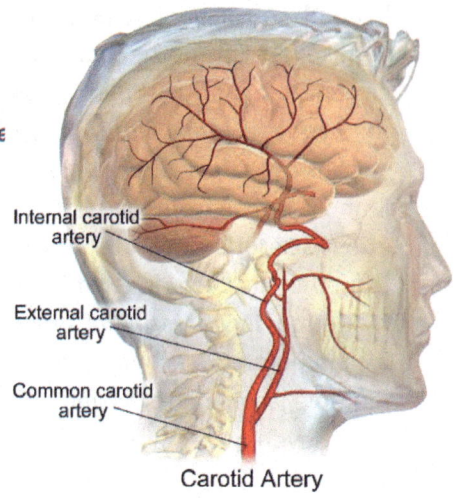

'Carotid arteries'. Medical gallery of Blausen Medical 2014. CC BY 3.0.

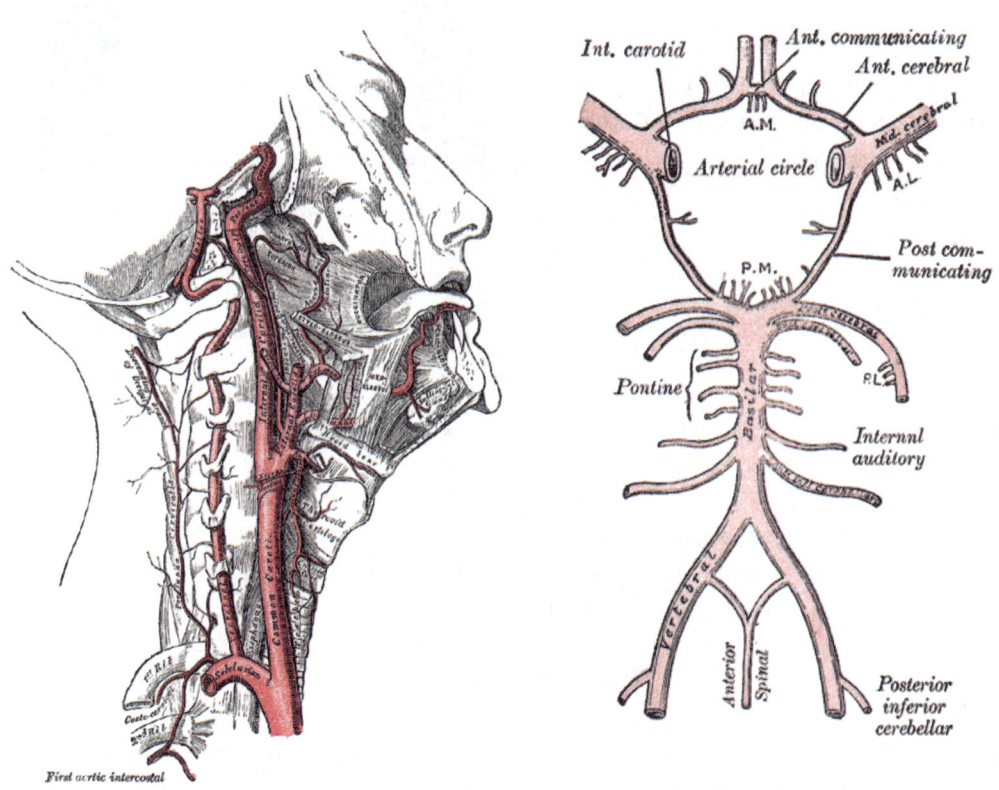

'The internal carotid in vertebral arteries'. Right Side. Henry Van Dyke Carter. Anatomy of the Human Body 1918 (Gray's Anatomy). Public domain.

'Circle of Willis'. Henry Van Dyke Carter. Anatomy of the Human Body 1918 (Gray's Anatomy). Public domain.

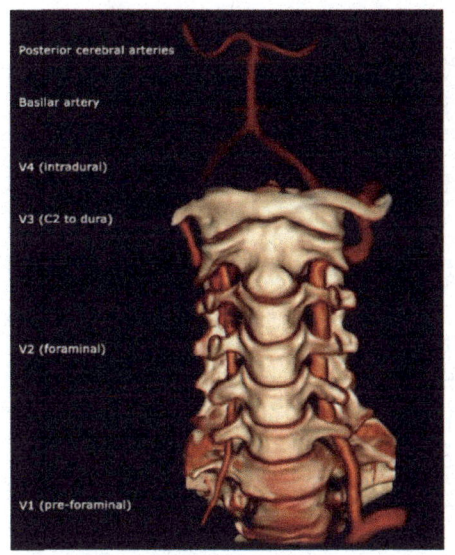

'Vertebral artery based upon 3D surface rendered CTA'. Frank Gaillard, own work. BY-SA 3.0.

The paired **vertebral arteries** connect the base of the brainstem and form the basilar artery. The basilar artery then connects back to the Circle of Willis. Occlusion of the basilar artery can lead to a fatal stroke due to the destruction of a significant portion of the brainstem or, in some cases, it can also lead to catastrophic locked-in syndrome, in which the patient is completely paralyzed, with the exception of vertical eye movement. The popular book and later on the film, *The Diving Bell and the Butterfly*, was written by French writer and editor of Elle magazine Jean-Dominique Bauby. He was able to write his final book using only eye blinks to communicate as he had suffered a basilar artery stroke and the resultant locked-in syndrome.

Atherosclerosis is the most common disease affecting the major arteries for the brain, carotid and vertebral arteries. Atherosclerosis refers to the gradual degeneration of the artery wall as a result of the accumulation of cholesterol. Beginning in adolescence, cholesterol gradually penetrates and accumulates in the middle lining of arteries. It particularly affects larger arteries. The reason due to which cholesterol accumulates is not well understood. Inheritance seems to be a significant factor, but the accumulation is also rapidly increased by high levels of

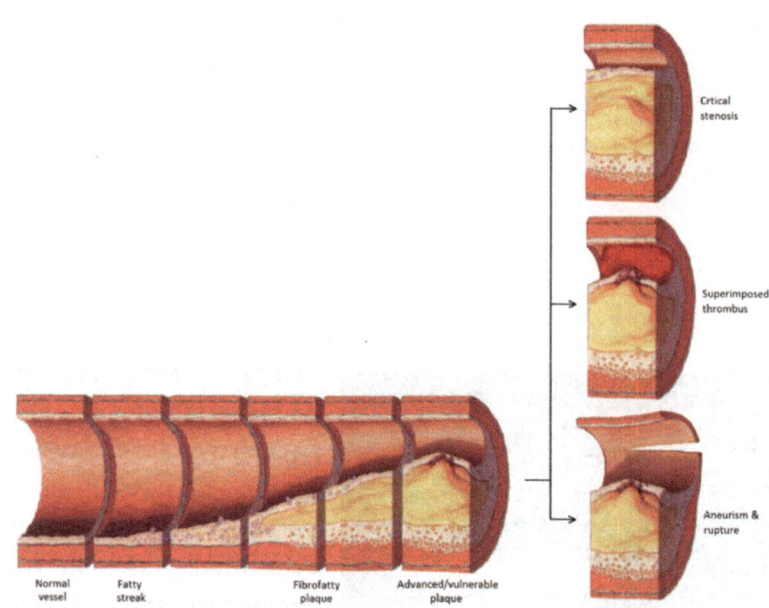

'Late complications of atherosclerosis'. Npatchett.CC BY-SA 4.0.

cholesterol in the bloodstream, high blood pressure, diabetes and tobacco use. Autopsy studies conducted in adolescents who died by trauma or young soldiers who died in combat demonstrate that this process starts very early in life but is significantly more rapid in those with even mild hypertension, mildly elevated glucose levels or cholesterol levels. Tobacco use is another primary factor. This is why emphasis on teaching young people about healthy life style choices is a central objective of Primary Stroke Prevention.

However, other conditions can also affect these arteries, such as **arterial dissections**. Artery walls contain three layers that resemble the layers of rubber seen if you cut a garden hose. If a tear occurs in the inner thin layer, blood can be forced in between the inner and middle layer creating a sort of blood blister or dissection. Dissections can completely occlude the artery or can extend for great lengths along an artery. Arteries with dissections become inflamed, and quite often, a clot or thrombus forms next to the damaged vessel wall. These clots can detach and float up into the brain and occlude smaller but critical arteries leading to strokes. Dissections tend to occur in carotid arteries or

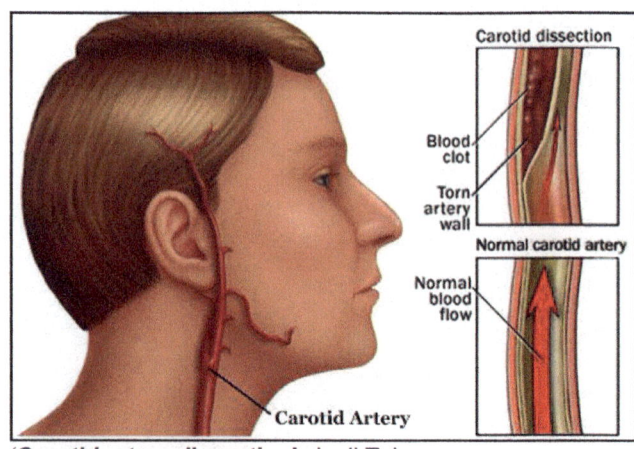

'Carotid artery dissection'. Junji Takano. www.homeopathyhome.com/forums forum/holistic-therapies/discussion/12520- the-magic-bullet-for-treating-stroke- fast-chart?t=12231

in the upper vertebral arteries. Minor trauma to the neck can be the primary cause of dissections. Auto accidents, sports activities, aggressive chiropractic adjustments or even turning one's neck to look at traffic behind one are all known causes of dissection.

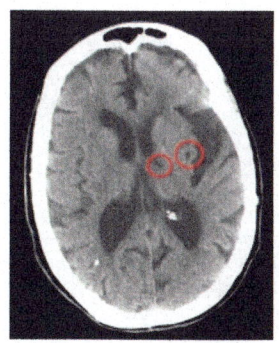

'Lacunar strokes'. Mikael Haggstrom. CC-BY-SA-3.0.

Much of the cerebral hemispheres and the brainstem receive blood supply by small artery branches coming from the larger arteries. The small arteries are known by several names such as the lenticulostriate arteries, depending on their location. These small arteries are greatly affected by hypertension as well as diabetes and age. The stress created by high blood pressure leads to gradual weakening and deterioration of the small vessel wall. This signifies the process of **arteriolosclerosis**, also referred to as lipohyalinosis. Eventually, small vessels may clot, producing a lacunar infarct, but the same disease process also weakens the vessel wall and can lead to bleeding. Therefore, the same disease can cause either an ischemic stroke or cerebral hemorrhage in the same patient. Less commonly, atherosclerosis from cholesterol accumulation or emboli can cause strokes through small arteries.

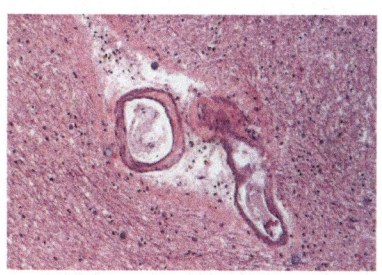

'Cerebral arteriolosclerosis (microangiopathy), damage of arterioles due to chronic arterial hypertension (high blood pressure)'. Patho-own work. CC-BY-SA 3.0.

As mentioned earlier, several strokes are not caused by disease in the arteries but are a result of an embolus originating from the heart or other sites in the body. Atrial fibrillation is the most common heart condition that leads to strokes due to embolus. In this condition, the upper chambers of the heart, the right and left atrium begin to quiver rather than pump blood into the ventricles. A patient may not notice this quivering effect or the **atrial fibrillation** may come and go for short intervals. Sometimes, a patient may develop a rapid heart rate or feel a fluttering or palpitation in their chest. Most of the times, there are no symptoms. The result of atrial fibrillation is that blood becomes stagnant inside the quivering atrium and forms clots. These clots are later ejected from the heart and may travel up to the main arteries of the brain causing a stroke. However, it is not clear how often atrial fibrillation causes strokes, but there are estimates that 20% to 30% of strokes are a result of atrial fibrillation. These strokes can almost be completely prevented by using anticoagulant drugs such as warfarin, also known as Coumadin. Newer high-priced drugs such as Eliquis and Xarelto are also highly effective.

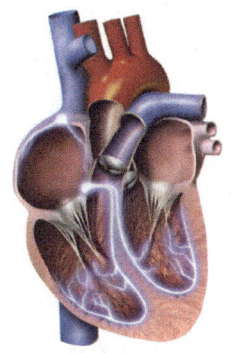
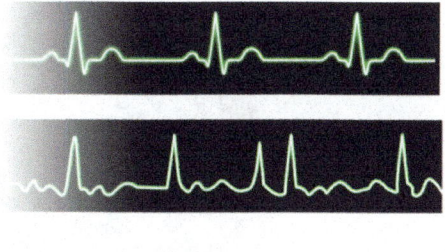

Atrial Fibrillation

'Atrial fibrillation'. BruceBlaus. CC BY-SA.

Other cardiac conditions that can lead to stroke include **patent foramen ovale,** but other less common conditions such as heart valve infections known as endocarditis or ventricular thrombus from clots forming on heart muscle tissue damage from a previous heart attack can also be responsible.

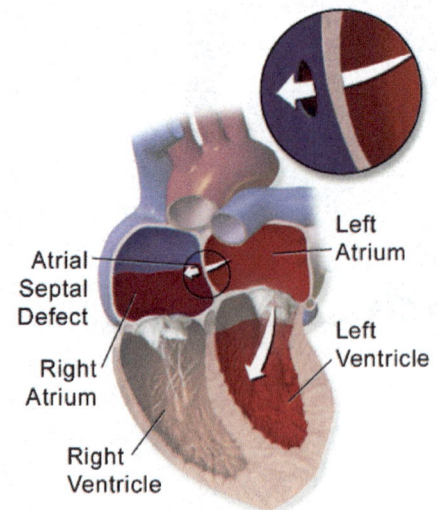

'Patent foramen ovale (atrial septal defect)'. Medical Gallery of Blausen Medical 2014. CC BY 3.0.

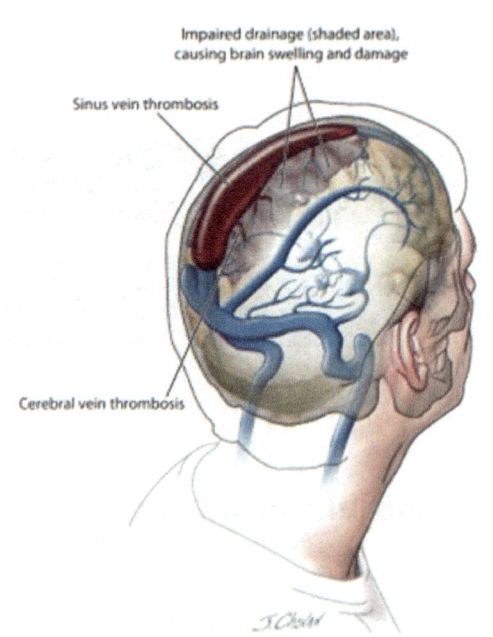

The least commonly encountered type stroke, which can also be quite fatal, is related to clotting of veins which drain blood away from the brain. Clotting in the draining veins is often referred to as **cerebral venous sinus thrombosis**. Venous sinus thrombosis is usually caused by diseases different from those affecting the arteries. Blood clotting disorders and infection are among the numerous disorders that can cause venous thrombosis. The effect can be strokes or hemorrhages or dangerous elevation of pressure inside the skull related to swelling and vessel engorgement due to the impaired venous drainage.

'Sinus and cerebral brain thrombosis'. Joe Chovan, medical illustrator. clotconnect.wpcomstaging.com/2011/02/07/sinus-and- cerebral- vein- thrombosis/

Finally, there are several rare blood disorders that can lead to clot formation and strokes. One of the most common causes of stroke on earth is sickle cell disease.

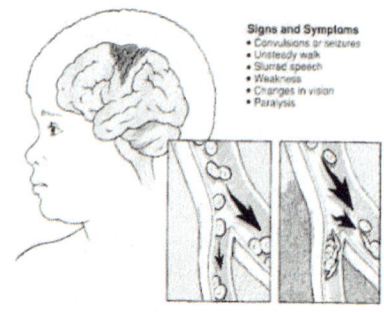

'Sickle cell and stroke'. sicklecell-ourvoice.blogspot.com/2009/06/sickle-cell-and-stroke.html

Chapter 2. TIAs

Stroke is the fifth leading cause of death in the United States and is the greatest cause of disability. Many patients at risk for stroke will experience warning symptoms or **transient ischemic attacks (TIA)**. TIA was originally defined as a sudden onset of loss of function of a segment of the brain lasting for less than 24 hours, brought on by a transient decrease in blood supply, which renders the brain ischemic in the area producing the symptom. Since the brain performs numerous different functions through various areas of the brain, there is a huge variety of TIA symptoms.

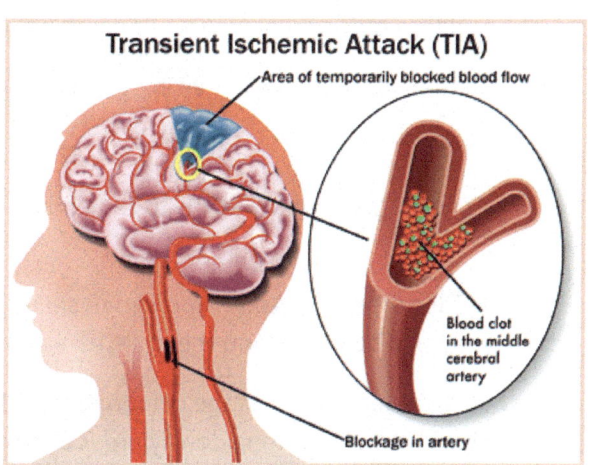

'Transient Ischemic attack'. https://i0.wp.com/a-fib.com/wp-content/uploads/2019/04/Transient-Ischemic-Attack-TIA-with-CU-400-x-300-min.png?w=400&ssl+1.CC BY-SA 4.0.

TIAs are produced by the same issue that causes strokes. A TIA is an important warning that somebody may be at risk for stroke, particularly in the first two weeks. The risk of stroke after transient ischemic attack is somewhere between 2% and 17% within the first 90 days. One study found that out of all ischemic strokes occurring within 30 days after the first TIA, 42% occurred within the first 24 hours. A total of 12%–30% of stroke patients have experienced a TIA before. A quarter of these TIAs occurred immediately prior to the stroke. However, it is important to note that TIAs are actually quite common and many people continue to lead normal lives and do not suffer a stroke after experiencing a TIA. After the first two weeks of TIA, the annual stroke risk is 3%–4%; TIA patients have different levels of risk, varying from low to very high. An estimated 240,000 TIAs are diagnosed each year in the USA. Probably another 300,000–700,000 cases are never reported. Therefore, the trick is to decide whether the TIA was an indication of an underlying disease process and if this indicates that the person has stroke risk factors that are not being addressed. Immediate medical intervention may reduce stroke risk by 80%.

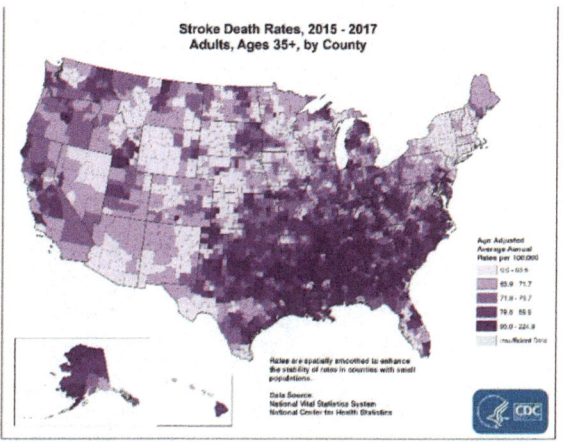

National Center for Chronic Disease Prevention and Health Promotion, Division of Heart Disease and Stroke Prevention.

Symptoms of TIA occur suddenly and are always temporary. They usually disappear in 10 to 20 minutes. TIA symptoms are similar to stroke symptoms. They vary depending on which part of the brain is affected. Common symptoms of TIA may include:

- Sudden numbness, tingling, weakness or loss of movement in one's face, arm or leg, especially on only one side of the body.

- Sudden vision changes.
- Sudden trouble in speaking.
- Sudden confusion or trouble understanding simple statements.
- Sudden problems with walking or balance.

Everyone should learn what **FAST** is to remember and recognize the following signs and symptoms of stroke:

- **F**. Face drooping. Ask the person to smile, and see if one side is drooping. One side of the face may also be numb, and the smile may appear uneven.
- **A**. Arm weakness. Ask the person to raise both arms. Is there weakness or numbness on one side? One arm drifting downward is a sign of one-sided arm weakness.
- **S**. Speech difficulty. People having a stroke may slur or have trouble speaking at all. Speech may be incomprehensible. Ask the person to repeat a simple sentence and look for any speech abnormalities.
- **T**. Time to call 9-1-1! If a person shows any of the symptoms above, even if the symptoms go away, call 9-1-1 and get the person to a hospital immediately.

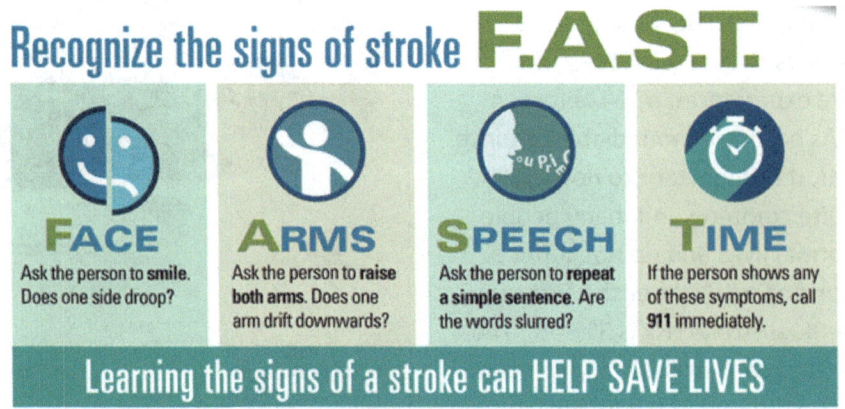

.cdc.gov/vitalsigns/stroke/index.html

TIAs, like strokes, can occur through a variety of mechanisms.

These include:

- **Low-flow TIAs**. Large artery low-flow TIAs are usually caused by gait narrowing or stenosis of the large arteries due to atherosclerotic buildup within the vessel wall. These areas of narrowing typically occur where blood flow is turbulent. The lower aspect of the internal carotid artery is a relatively common area for this to occur. It also happens in other areas such as the middle cerebral artery or basilar artery. Remarkably, low-flow TIAs are not nearly as common as embolic TIAs. The reason for this is that as atherosclerotic buildup happens over the years, the body can often create alternate blood flow patterns or collateral blood flow to compensate.

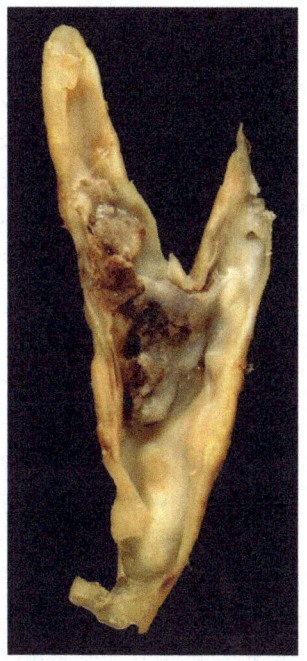

'Carotid plaque'. By Ed Uthman, CC BY 2.0, https://commons.wikimedia.org/w/index.php?curid=1208790

- **Embolic TIA**. Embolic TIAs are characterized by discrete, usually single, more prolonged (hours) episodes of focal neurologic symptoms. The most common source of embolic TIAs is the formation of clots or thrombus on the inflamed or ulcerated surface of atherosclerotic arteries. These clots will detach and travel, occluding smaller arteries supplying the brain. Similar to low-flow TIAs, atherosclerotic buildup is usually found in large arteries which have turbulent blood flow. The carotid artery, the aorta and several other smaller arteries can create this complication. Emboli can also perform in the heart. Atrial fibrillation is the most common cause but emboli traveling to a patent foramen ovale or coming off a sick left ventricle or abnormal heart valve are other possibilities. If the primary pathologic process is considered to be embolic, a diligent search for its source is necessary before therapy to prevent future stroke is initiated.

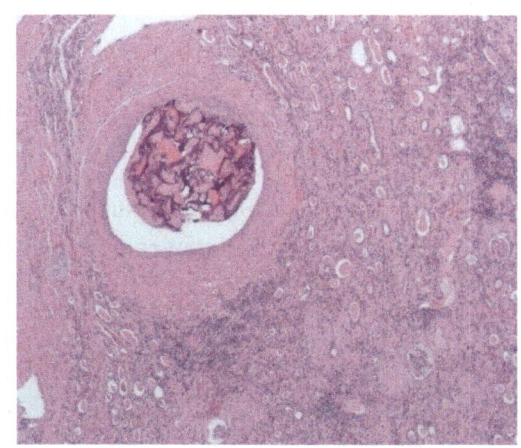

'Embolus within large artery'. By Nephron, own work, CC BY-SA 3.0, https://commons.wikimedia.org/w/index.php?curid=5877793

- **Lacunar** or **small vessel TIA** — Lacunar or penetrating or small vessel TIAs are caused by transient cerebral ischemia induced by stenosis of one of the intracerebral penetrating vessels arising from the middle cerebral artery or the basilar artery.

Occasionally, recurrent stereotyped TIAs occur; in this case, the term lacunar or small vessel TIAs seems appropriate. Lacunar or small vessel TIAs are considered to be caused either by degeneration of these small blood vessels due to the effect of long-standing high blood pressure, diabetes or age. Less commonly, lacunar infarcts can occur due to atherosclerotic obstructive lesions at the origin of the penetrating artery.

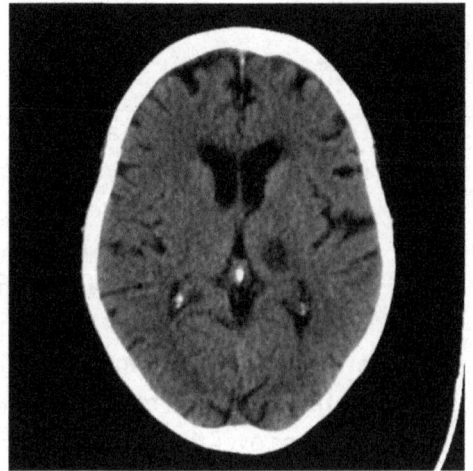

'*Lacunar infarct*'. Case courtesy of Dr David Cuete, <a href="https://radiopaedia.org/">Radiopaedia.org</a>. From the case <a href="https://radiopaedia.org/cases/36507">rID: 36507</a>. CC BY-NC-SA 3.0.

It is important to note that it is not entirely unusual for somebody to experience recurrent episodes of brain symptoms suggesting TIA actually due to other conditions. Distinguishing between true TIAs and TIA imitating other conditions requires evaluation by a physician, experienced with TIA and stroke, as well as diagnostic testing. Some other conditions that can imitate TIAs include:

- Epileptic seizures. Partial seizures are epileptic events arising from a small area of the brain which can cause focal brain symptoms without creating a convulsion.
- Migraine auras.
- Syncope/fainting.
- Vertigo due to inner ear problems which can cause transient episodic dizziness.
- Pressure- or position-related peripheral nerve or nerve root compression that causes transient paresthesia and numbness.
- Metabolic perturbations such as hypoglycemia and hepatic, renal, and pulmonary encephalopathies that can produce temporary aberrations in behavior and movement.
- Transient global amnesia.
- Intracranial hemorrhage.

The following are indications that neurologic symptoms may not be due to true TIAs or strokes:

- Gradual build-up of symptoms (more than five minutes)

- Advance of symptoms from one body part to another (without passing the midline)
- Progression of symptoms from one type to another
- Isolated disturbance of vision in both eyes characterized by the occurrence of positive phenomena
- Isolated sensory symptoms with remarkable focal distribution, such as in a finger, chin or tongue
- Very brief spells (less than 30 seconds)
- Identical spells occurring over a period of more than one year
- Isolated brainstem symptoms, such as dysarthria, diplopia or hearing loss.

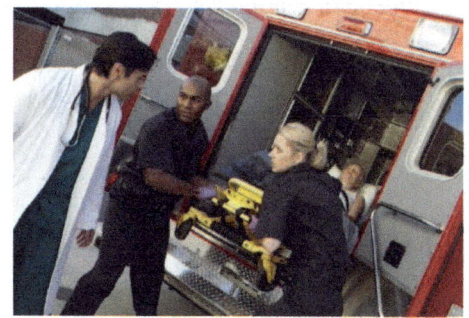

cdc.gov/stroke/treatments.htm

The occurrence of a TIA should trigger immediate referral to the emergency department or a clinic equipped to perform a comprehensive TIA or stroke evaluation. Since the evaluation usually includes rapidly obtaining laboratory exams, heart tests and brain imaging studies, this usually requires an evaluation in a hospital emergency department. If the emergency department physician decides that the symptoms may be related to a TIA or stroke, an evaluation to screen for multiple stroke possibilities will begin. Stroke risk factors will be assessed and addressed. Typically, medications are prescribed to reduce the likelihood of thrombosis depending on the mechanism suspected. Treatment is discussed in further detail in Chapter 6.

The following tests should be considered immediately:

- CBC or blood count.
- PT, PTT which are tests of coagulation.
- Electrolytes, creatinine and glucose. Low glucose and high glucose closely levels can cause brain malfunction that can imitate TIAs or stroke.
- Lipids. LDL cholesterol may be checked even when the patient is nonfasting.
- Immediate brain and vascular imaging. This ordinarily comprises brain CT with CT angiogram. Ruling out carotid artery stenosis is a high priority.
- EKG to assess for atrial fibrillation or myocardial infarction.

Brain imaging with MRI also has an important role in evaluating TIA. Since MRI usually cannot be performed immediately, a brain CT and CT angiogram are conducted as the initial imaging studies. Brain MRI studies also include a sequence referred to as **diffusion weighted imaging** or **DWI**.

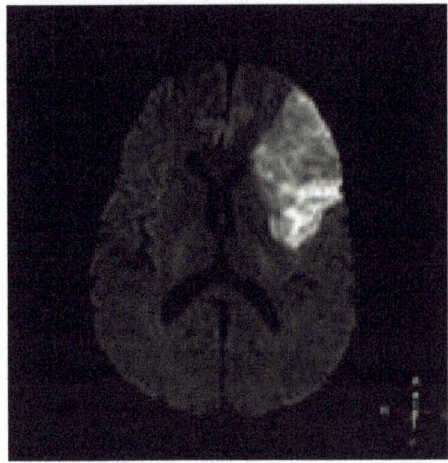

'Ischemic stroke'
radiopaedia.org/articles/ischaemic-stroke. CC BY-NC-SA 3.0.

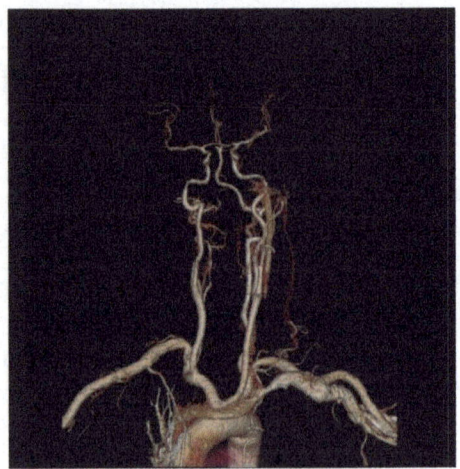

'CT angiogram of cervical arteries, reconstruction view'.
https://radiopaedia.org/articles/ct-angiography-of-the-cerebral-arteries?lang=us. CC BY-NC-SA 3.0.

Small areas of infarction can often be seen for 72 hours after resolution of TIA symptoms. Patients with abnormalities on DWI have a significantly higher risk of stroke compared to patients with normal MRI studies. Risk for early stroke for TIA patients with a normal MRI may be as low as 0.4%. An abnormal DWI study raises stroke risk 20-fold.

Furthermore, the distribution of the DWI abnormality allows the physician to guess the mechanism of the TIA or stroke. Different patterns of DWI correlate with a variety of different diseases such as embolism or lacunar infarction.

Cardiac monitoring is an essential part of evaluation to exclude atrial fibrillation in the context of embolic TIA or stroke. Cardiac rhythm monitoring with inpatient telemetry, outpatient Ziopatch or Holter monitor is useful for patients without a clear etiology after initial brain imaging and electrocardiography.

Whether hospitalization is required for TIA evaluation is not clear, but urgent assessment and management are essential regardless of inpatient or outpatient status.

The **ABCD2 score** (for Age, Blood pressure, Clinical features, Duration of symptoms, and Diabetes) is a prognostic assessment tool designed to identify patients at high risk of ischemic stroke in the first two days following TIA. Although 2009 AHA/ASA guidelines advocated the use of ABCD2 score, subsequent studies found that the score does not provide an accurate estimate of stroke risk and clinical decisions based on an ABCD2 score cut-off are subject to significant misclassification error.

Risk stratification for TIA with ABCD2 score

ABCD²	Criteria	Points
Age	≥ 60 years	1
Blood pressure	≥140/80	1
Clinical features	Unilateral weakness	2
	Speech impairment without weakness	1
Duration of Sx	>60 minutes	2
	10-59 minutes	1
Diabetes	Yes	1

Score	2day-risk for stroke	Recurrence within 90days
0-3	Low	1.0%
4-5	Moderate	4.1%
6-7	High	8.1%

JAMA 2000;284:2901-2906

ABCD2-I	Points
ABCD2 +	7

I = (image)
  MRI : acute infarction on DWI
  CT : acute or old infarction
	3

Stroke 2010;41:1907-13

'ABCD2 Score for TIA'. http://www.emdocs.net/8538-2/. CC BY 4.0.

Chapter 3. Recognition of Stroke Symptoms and Need for Immediate Response

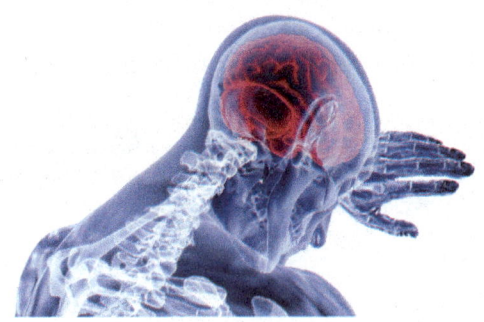

By VSRao. Pixabay

- Each year, approximately 795,000 people suffer a stroke. About 600,000 of these are first attacks, and 185,000 are recurrent attacks.[1]

- Stroke is the third leading cause of death in the United States. More than 140,000 people die each year from stroke in the United States.[2] It accounted for nearly one of every 17 deaths in the United States in 2006.

- On an average, someone in the United States has a stroke every 40 seconds.[2]

- Nearly three-quarters of all strokes occur in people aged over 65. The risk of having a stroke more than doubles each decade after the age of 55.

- Strokes can and do occur at ANY age. Nearly one fourth of all strokes occur in people under the age of 65.

- Among stroke survivors, many face serious disability for the remainder of their life. Stroke is the leading cause of serious, long-term disability in the United States.[1]

A 2003 study in Massachusetts found that 80% of average citizens would call 911 if they thought someone was having a stroke or heart attack but only 18% of adults were aware about the signs and symptoms of stroke.[3]

---

[1] Benjamin EJ, Blaha MJ, Chiuve SE, et al. on behalf of the American Heart Association Statistics Committee and Stroke Statistics Subcommittee. Heart disease and stroke statistics—2017 update: a report from the American Heart Association. *Circulation*. 2017;135:e229–e445.

[2] Vital Signs: Recent trends in stroke death rates – United States, 2000–2015. MMWR 2017;66.

[3] Addressing Stroke Signs and Symptoms Through Public Education: The Stroke Heroes Act FAST Campaign Hilary K Wall, MPH, Brianne M Beagan, MPH, H June O'Neill, MPH, Kathleen M Foell, RD, MS, and Cynthia L Boddie-Willis, MD, MPH Prev Chronic Dis. 2008 Apr; 5(2): A49.

A typical stroke can result in the death of brain cells at a rate of 1.9 million cells per minute with the loss of blood flow.[4] Now, with the advent of thrombolytic therapy (TPA) and thrombectomy (clot retrieval), there is a way to halt this process and save the brain. However, it is a race against time. TPA can be administered only up to 4.5 hours after the onset of stroke symptoms. Even then, it is evidently significantly more effective if delivered within minutes rather than hours after the appearance of symptoms. After 4.5 hours, the risk of fatal brain hemorrhage outweighs any possible small benefit.

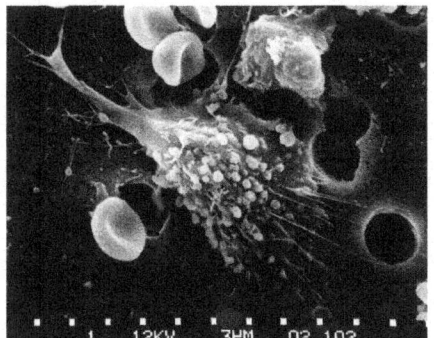

'Cell Death'. By Susan Arnold (photographer). Public Domain.

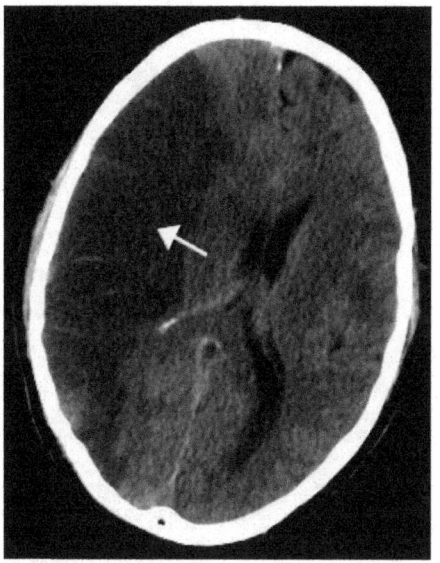

Thrombectomy can be performed beyond 4.5 hours and can still result in good outcomes, but stroke victims clearly have a considerably better chance of a good recovery if they receive treatment within 90 minutes compared to several hours later. This makes every second crucial. Multiple small delays over trivial details often cause serious delay in treatment. This is why excellent communication and coordination between all medical personnel involved in initial stroke care is significant.

'CT of the brain withan MCA infarct'. By INFARCT.jpg: Lucien Monfilsderivative work: Suraj - INFARCT.jpg, CC BY-SA 3.0, https://commons.wikimedia.org/w/index.php

However, the biggest delay usually occurs before 911 is called. People who suffer strokes are commonly unaware about what has transpired. Part of this lack of insight is due to the effect of the stroke on brain recognition. The person may have complete paralysis of one side but the part of the brain that should recognize the problem might also be affected. We call this **agnosia** or "**neglect**". The stroke patient may not even recognize that their paralyzed arm even belongs to them. And therefore, the natural response might be for the stroke victim to remain in bed or in their chair or even on the floor until they are discovered. People who live alone may be discovered on the floor days after their stroke occurred. Even if the person is aware that there is a problem, they will often insist on going to bed to try to sleep it off. Therefore, it is necessary that their companions, family, coworkers and any bystander be aware of the signs of stroke and know to call 911 immediately. This is one of the primary missions of SAO, to teach everyone about stroke recognition and to understand they need to call 911.

---

[4] Time Is Brain—Quantified
Jeffrey L Saver
Stroke. 2006;37:263–266

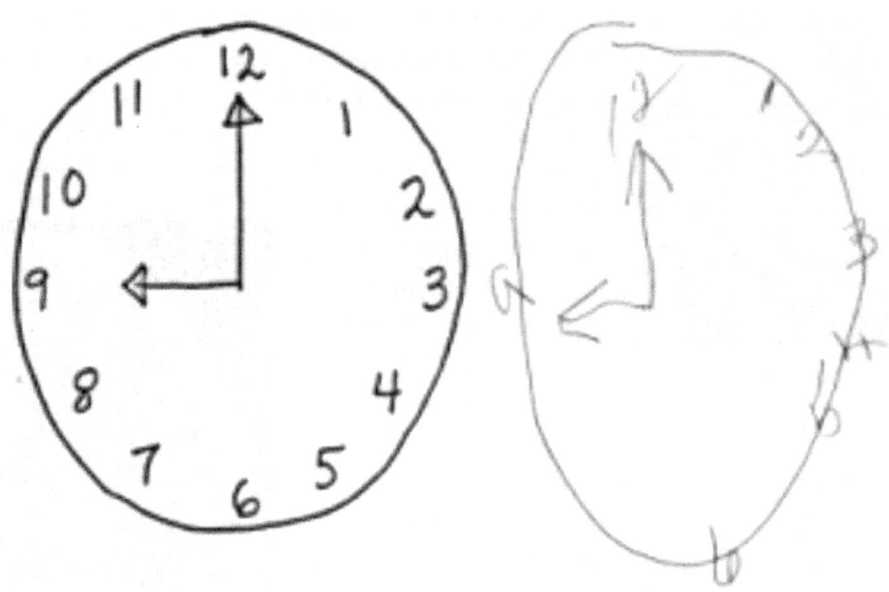

Unilateral neglect during clock drawing. The example is shown above and the patient's copy to the right. Not uncommonly, patients with left neglect sketch the entire circle and write the numerals 12, 3, 6, and 9 at their correct locations. The patient was satisfied that she had sketched the entire clock face shown to her. She acknowledged her omissions when they were indicated to her. Note the bunching of numerals on the right side, another characteristic of clock drawing by patients with neglect.

'Unilateral neglect during clock drawing'. Mark, Victor. (2003). Acute versus chronic functional aspects of unilateral spatial neglect. Frontiers in bioscience : a journal and virtual library. 8. e172-89. 10.2741/973.

There are a number of methods to teach people regarding the symptoms of stroke. SAO recommends teaching **FAST**.

F-Face. Do you see any asymmetry on the concerned person's face? Asking them to smile or frown may help bring this out. One side of the face may have a reduced normal fold between the nose and corner of the mouth, known as flattening of the nasolabial fold. Typically though, the patient's forehead is not affected by stroke.

A-Arm. Is there weakness in one arm? Asking them to raise both arms quickly together may bring out any subtle weakness. The weak arm will react slower. Perhaps the patient is unable to keep the arm elevated at shoulder level or even raise it at all. Typically, the patient's hand is also affected, thus they have a weak grip or cannot perform fast finger tapping like they can with the other hand.

S-Speech. Speech can be affected in multiple ways. The stroke victim may not be able to understand what is being said to them. They may not be able to name simple objects or even names of people. They may understand that they cannot reply in a comprehensible manner. Sometimes, their speech might just be slurred. The best way to screen for speech changes is to ask the patient to repeat an easily spoken phrase. They must repeat it exactly with no slurring, without dropping any words. For example, ask them to say "I live in Oregon" or "the sky is blue". They should be able to say every word perfectly. If not, speech change from stroke can be suspected.

T-Time. Call 911 immediately. This is always better than driving to the hospital even if you live across the street. As soon as the EMS first responders arrive, they can notify the emergency department so that the entire stroke team is mobilized prior to the patient's arrival. Do not give aspirin because there is no way to determine whether the stroke is due to a blockage of blood flow or hemorrhage in the brain.

Many stroke centers prefer to use the acronym **BEFAST**. This includes:

B-Balance. Sudden dizziness, loss of balance or coordination.

E-Eyes. Some trouble seeing from one or both eyes.

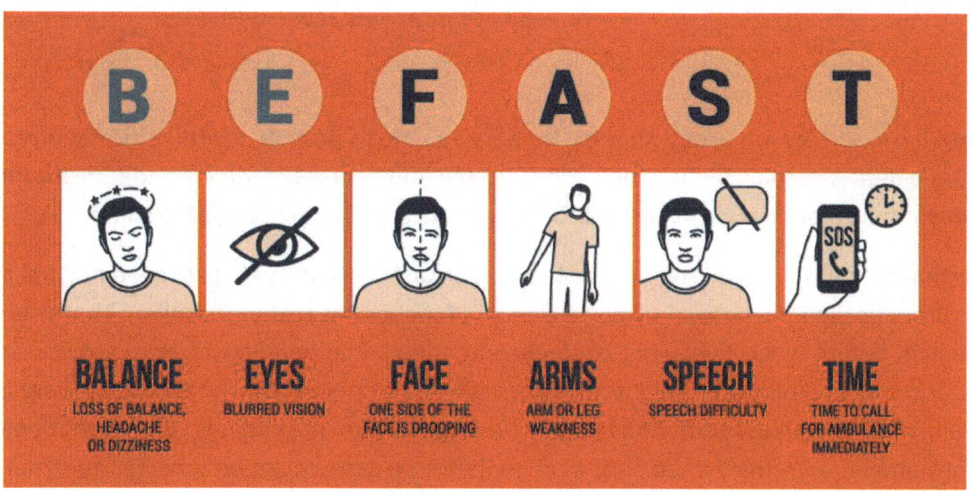

'BEFAST'. Thaihealth.or.th. CC BY-NC-SA 3.0 TH.

SAO has opted to use **FAST** with the belief that it can be remembered by a greater number of people.

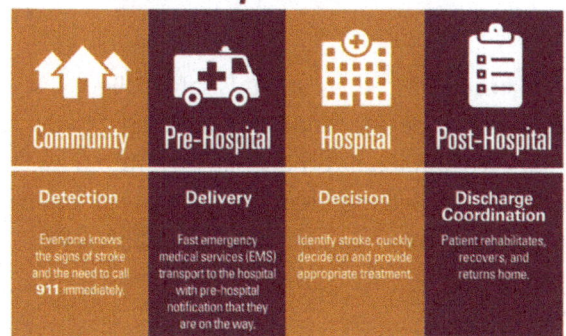

cdc.gov/vitalsigns/stroke/index.html

Calling 911 by telephone is the most effective and the preferred way of accessing the local **emergency medical services** or **EMS**. Calling the stroke victim's doctor or calling a nurse advice line can lead to a loss of valuable minutes. Calling 911 will connect you with the local EMS dispatch office operator who will establish immediate contact with emergency responders. When calling from a landline, the dispatch operator can usually map the calling telephone number to an address in a database. But nowadays, over 80% of phone calls to 911 occur with cell phones which do not allow this option. The dispatch operator will need to know the location of the stroke victim; therefore, it is necessary that the caller be able to provide an address or details about the location.

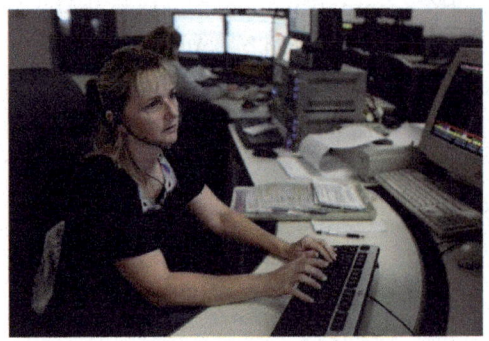
'Dispatch operator'. Public Domain.

The dispatch operator may wish for the caller to remain on the line in order to provide additional directions. The operator will have questions. Is the patient breathing or breathless? Are they conscious? Do they have chest pain? At the same time, the stroke victim still requires close observation. The **ABCs** (airway, breathing, circulation) need to be remembered as well. Ordinarily, the stroke victim just needs to be kept in a safe position until EMS responders arrive; however, significantly, the bystander may require to be ready to intervene, even with CPR.

Furthermore, it is also very important that bystanders be able to provide useful information to the EMS providers. Basic details such as the person's identity, age and general medical condition are important. Further relevant information such as pregnancy or recent surgeries are crucial to share.

- A highly critical question is when was the person last seen normal? **Last seen normal** means the last time the victim was awake and talking and functioning at their baseline. That could mean the night before when they went to sleep. Sometimes, the person will get up to use the bathroom in the middle the night; however, we do not necessarily know if they were thinking or talking normally unless somebody actually engaged them in a conversation at that point. This information is extremely important to know before a patient can be qualified for treatment of TPA or thrombectomy.

- Another important question is whether the victim is taking any blood thinners? Drugs like Coumadin/warfarin, apixaban/Eliquis, rivaroxaban/Xarelto or Pradaxa are powerful anticoagulant blood thinners. If the person was taking one of these anticoagulant drugs and received TPA unknowingly, the risk of serious intracranial bleeding is nearly 30%.

- Families and bystanders can also help by collecting the victim's medication bottles or providing a medication list to give to the EMS responder.

When the EMS responders arrive, they must move quickly to ensure that the patient is safe, collect necessary information and then communicate back to the dispatch operators and the receiving emergency department. All EMS personnel go through extensive training, but there can be differences in the level of training. In remote areas, the ambulance service may be dependent on volunteer firemen while trained paramedics are usually available in cities. Central Oregon has a combination of different types of ambulance services.

The American Heart Association policy recommendations for EMS include:

- Support ABCs: airway, breathing, circulation and provide oxygen if required.

- Perform pre-hospital stroke assessments, usually BEFAST and C-STAT.

- Establish the time when the patient was last normal.
- Rapid transportation to the nearest Primary Stroke Center, Comprehensive Stroke Center or TPA capable hospital.
- EMS can opt to bypass a local hospital which does not possess the necessary stroke resources if the regional stroke center is within reasonable transport range.
- Send an alert to the receiving hospital as soon as possible about the potential stroke patient. In Central Oregon, this step is called activation of **STROKE ONE**.
- Check the patient's glucose level if possible.

EMS responders must make a quick assessment to determine if the victim is displaying symptoms of stroke. They may use FAST or BEFAST. The idea is that they are not attempting to make a specific diagnosis but rather to identify anyone who might possibly need urgent treatment for stroke even if the patient may have a different medical problem. This can be a challenge because patients may be experiencing multiple problems simultaneously. Severe bloodstream infection, sepsis, can be accompanied by stroke. Stroke victims who are found down after a long period of time usually also have other serious medical problems that develop due to their immobility. Once the EMS responder has determined that the patient may have

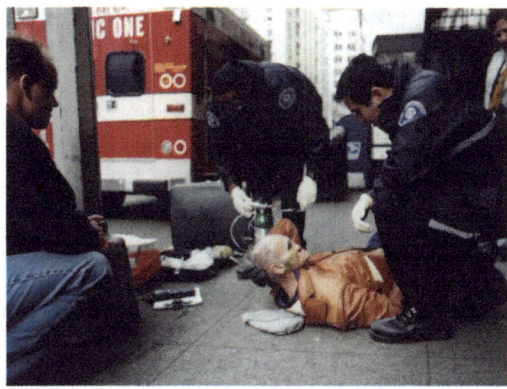

'Man having stroke'. By Joe Goldberg. flickr.com/photos/goldberg/43951184 CC BY-SA 2.0

suffered a stroke, the responder will contact the dispatch operator and the receiving emergency department and announce that they will be transporting a patient as **STROKE ONE**.

BE FAST Stroke Screen (Balance - Eyes - Face - Arm - Speech - Time)	Normal	Abnormal	
Balance-Finger to nose, gait test Normal: Not dizzy, steady gait Abnormal: Inability to walk, abnormal gait, ataxia	Normal	Balance	Gait/Ataxia
Eyes-Visual Acuity, visual field assessment Normal: Vision normal for patient, with or without correction Abnormal: Sudden double or blurred vision, blindness, visual field cut	Normal	Left	Right
Face-Have patient smile or show teeth Normal: Both sides of face move equally Abnormal: One side of face weak/unequal/movement absent	Normal	Left	Right
Arm-Arm-Extend arms, close eyes, palms down Normal: Both arms move equally or not at all Abnormal: One arm drifts compared to the other	Normal	Left	Right
Speech-Ask patient to repeat, "You can't teach an old dog new tricks" Normal: Patient uses correct words with no slurring Abnormal: Speech fluency disruption, slurred speech or is mute	Normal	Slurred	Fluency/Comprehension
Time- Onset and Last seen normal		Time	
New onset of neurologic deficit within the last 6 hours?		Yes	No
New onset of neurologic deficit within the last 24 hours?		Yes	No
If one or more components of the BE FAST Stroke Screen is abnormal and the patient was last seen normal < 24 hours prior to arrival, the stroke screen is considered POSITIVE. Continue to C-STAT evaluation.			

Almost all regions of the country also employ additional scoring systems to identify patients who have suffered large vessel occlusion strokes. These tools include RACE, LAMS or **C-STAT** (formerly CPSS). In

Central Oregon, EMS responders are trained to perform the **Cincinnati Stroke Triage Assessment Tool (C-STAT)**. It is a brief examination and screening technique that allows the identification of the majority of patients who have suffered the most serious strokes due to the occlusion of major cerebral arteries. These patients may have arterial clots that are too large to respond to TPA but can benefit from clot retrieval/thrombectomy if they arrive early enough at a hospital with thrombectomy capabilities. In Central Oregon, St. Charles Medical Center in Bend is the only hospital that can offer thrombectomy.

C-STAT includes only three quick examination parts.

- 2 points: Conjugate gaze deviation.

- 1 point: Cannot provide his/her age or current month and does not follow one of 2 commands (eye closure, opening and closing hand).

- 1 point: Cannot hold arm (either right or left) up for 10 seconds before arm falls to bed.

A C-STAT Score of 2 or more = high likelihood of large vessel occlusion stroke. Therefore, as patients are being transported to the emergency department, they will be designated as STROKE ONE and either C-STAT positive or C-STAT negative.

CINCINNATI STROKE TRIAGE ASSESSMENT TOOL - C-STAT		
	Points	Definition
GAZE		Unable to look in certain direction with both eyes.
Absent (Normal)	0	
Present (Abnormal)	2	
ARM WEAKNESS		Cannot hold up arm(s) for 10 seconds.
Absent (Normal)	0	
Present (Abnormal)	1	
LEVEL OF CONCSIOUSNESS		Incorrectly answers at least one of two LOC questions AND does not follow at least one of two commands.
Absent (Normal)	0	LOC Questions - What month is it? How old are you?
Present (Abnormal)	1	LOC Commands - Open your eyes. Make a fist.
C-STAT positive is defined as a score of ≥ 2		

In Central Oregon, we are attempting to implement a regional triage system for use by all EMS departments which ultimately refer to St. Charles in Bend. For patients who are C-STAT positive, the outcomes may be worse if they are transported to the wrong hospital, resulting in an even longer delay before they can undergo life-saving thrombectomy. For patients who with large vessel occlusion, the majority will benefit by direct transport to hospitals which can offer endovascular treatment. For Central Oregon, this means direct transport, often by air ambulance, to St. Charles in Bend.

Time of Onset/Last Normal	BE FAST	C-STAT	Action #1	Action #2
0-6 hours	Positive	Positive	Activate **STROKE 1**	Transport directly to **Bend**
0-6 hours	Positive	Negative	Activate **STROKE 1**	Transport to **closest facility**
6-24 hours	Positive	Positive	Activate **STROKE 1**	Transport directly to **Bend**
6-24 hours	Positive	Negative	Do Not Activate	Transport to **closest facility**
Unknown onset & Last Normal < 24 hours	Positive	Positive	Activate **STROKE 1**	Transport directly to **Bend**
Unknown onset & Last Normal < 24 hours	Positive	Negative	Do Not Activate	Transport to **closest facility**
*** Symptomatic and improving			Activate **STROKE 1**	As defined above
*** Complete resolution prior to arrival			Do Not Activate	Transport to **closest facility**

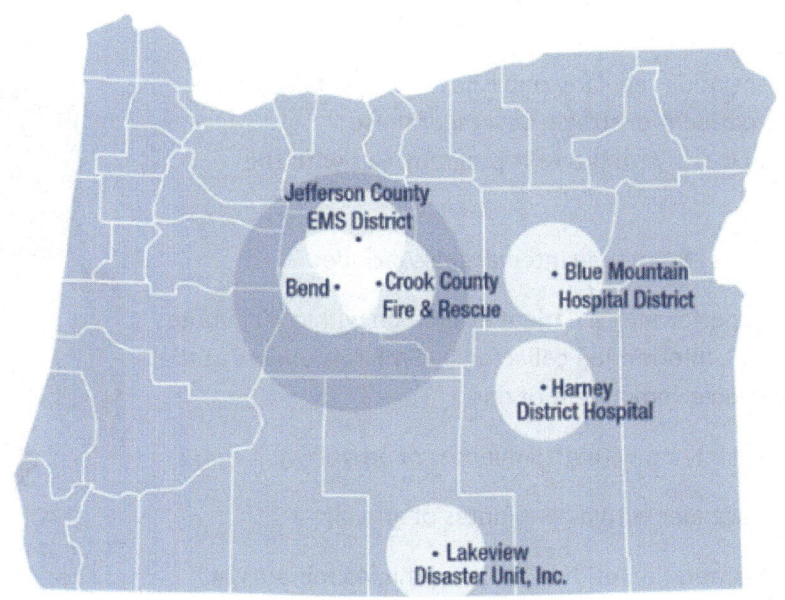

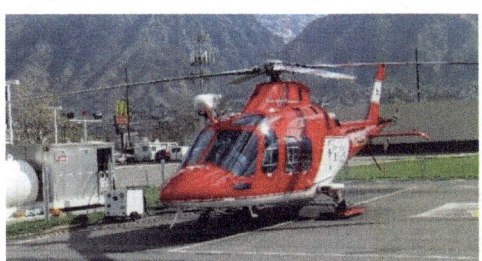

https://flickr.com/photos/88663091@N04/33797567125.CC BY-SA 2.0.

Air ambulance transport is extremely expensive. An unexpected helicopter trip from one side of the state to the other can cost up to $40,000. No one would ever want to be in the position of declining life-saving ambulance transport because it was unaffordable. SAO encourages everyone in Central Oregon to purchase inexpensive air ambulance insurance which typically costs less than $100 a year for a family.

For STROKE ONE patients, the emergency department would have already activated members of the stroke care team even before the patient arrives. There must be rapid and simultaneous communication between many healthcare professionals. This includes ED nurses, ED physicians, neurologists, CT scan technicians, radiologists, stroke interventionalists, laboratory technicians and EKG technicians. The goal is to make a decision about administering TPA within 60 minutes or preferably within 45 minutes. The second goal is to decide whether the patient should be taken to the radiology procedure room for possible thrombectomy/clot retrieval. Communication among so many people with such strict time requirements seems impossible but training and careful organization overcomes much of the difficulty. Currently, the system depends upon many phone calls, often going through the hospital communications operator. Bottlenecks can occur along any part of this complicated communication pathway. In the future, cloud-based secure texting may replace the need for so many phone calls.

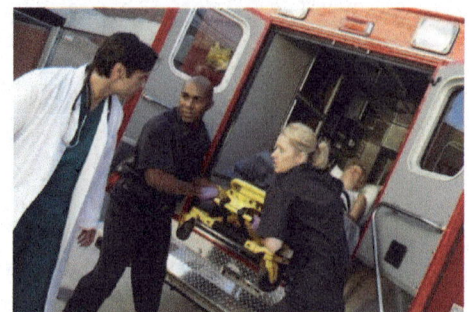

cdc.gov/stroke/treatments.htm

The American Heart Association regularly publishes research-based recommendations for treatment of stroke. Several of these recommendations are included with the AHA program, **Get with the Guidelines**.

The Get with the Guidelines stroke time interval goals include:

- The ED physician performing a patient evaluation within 10 minutes of arrival in the ED. Information collected by EMS responders at the scene is an invaluable component of this.

- Notifying the stroke team within 15 minutes of arrival.

- Reaching the CT scanner within 25 minutes of arrival.

- Radiologist's interpretation of the CT scan within 45 minutes of arrival.

- Goal is **door to needle time of** within 60 minutes for starting IV TPA.

- For thrombectomy eligible patients, the goal for **door to groin puncture time** is under 90 minutes.

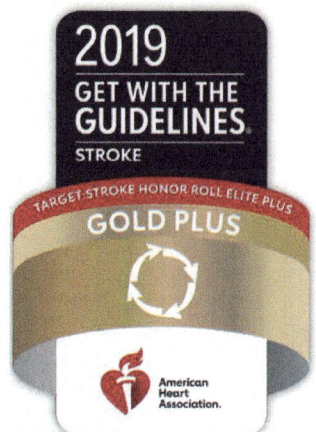

St. Charles Stroke Program has been awarded a Gold Plus designation for several years.

Hospitals may be certified by the Joint Commission, the largest national hospital accreditation organization, as Stroke Centers. The certification requirements are very strict and frequently monitored. There are different levels which include:

Comprehensive Stroke Center. This requires a 24/7 stroke team, dedicated neuro-intensive care, 24/7 neurosurgical care, extensive experience in managing subarachnoid hemorrhages and administration of IV thrombolytics. Currently, there are four hospitals in Oregon which are certified as comprehensive stroke centers. This includes OHSU, Providence St. Vincent, Legacy Emanuel and Riverbend Medical Center.

Thrombectomy Capable Stroke Center. This is a new designation that requires treatment with mechanical thrombectomy for at least 30 patients over 24 months. St. Charles in Bend may soon become eligible for this designation.

Primary Stroke Center. This designation acquires a 24/7 acute stroke team and 24/7 neurology or neurology telemedicine coverage, capability of treating with IV thrombolytics such as TPA, designated stroke beds and strict tracking and monitoring of performance measures. St. Charles Medical Center in Bend is the only primary stroke center in Central Oregon.

Acute Stroke Ready Hospital. This requires a dedicated stroke focus program with medical professionals trained in stroke care with the capability to perform CT imaging and administer TPA. They must also have transfer protocols in place for transferring to a PSC or CSC.

Technical advancements have rendered stroke care considerably more effective, but good stroke outcomes still require rapid recognition of stroke symptoms, fast transport of the patient and treatment within an extremely short period of time. However, none of our new medical technology will be helpful unless stroke victims and their families know how to recognize stroke and access the healthcare system immediately.

Chapter 4. Medical Therapies for Acute Stroke

When a patient with stroke reaches the hospital, several things need to be addressed quickly. Healthcare providers must ensure that the patient is breathing adequately, receiving sufficient oxygen and has a satisfactory blood pressure. A natural physiological response during stroke is extremely high

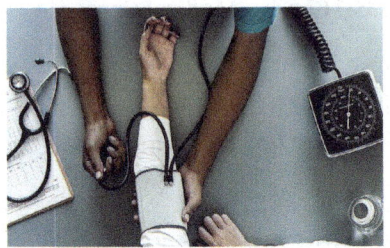
Courtesy Pickpik. Royalty free.

blood pressure. This is a neurological reflex that attempts to force more blood to the ischemic brain tissue. During the first 48 hours, doctors will allow the blood pressure to become very high, as much as 220/120, to enable the high blood pressure reflex to increase blood flow. This is known as **permissive hypertension**. Moreover, blood glucose levels must be higher than 60. High glucose levels may also be harmful, but strict treatment of lower glucose levels has not proven to be helpful.

Like complex, carefully engineered machines, several of the brains systems have redundancies. Therefore, if one area of the brain is destroyed, there may be other areas of brain tissue or extra neurons that can take over its function. With stroke, numerous brain cells die quickly but others become sick and quit functioning while still being capable of recovering if blood supply is restored fast. Furthermore, neurons do not necessarily die immediately. They can actually die slowly over several days. During this period of slow neuron death, multiple abnormal processes occur simultaneously. This includes **no reflow phenomena** wherein blood vessels stop blood flow even after blood pressure is restored. **Excitotoxic neurotransmitters**, such as NMDA, are chemicals normally used by neurons to communicate with other brain cells. But, when NMDA is released by brain cells damaged by ischemia in massive quantities, it causes other brain cells to get fired electrically, out-of-control, and burn themselves out. Moreover, brain cell membranes lose their electrical charge and allow toxic calcium ions to enter the cell and damage the mitochondria which are important energy plants for cell function. Something happens to the cell's DNA leading it to malfunction and turn on genes that will

'NDMA receptor which becomes overstimalated by excitotoxic neurotransmitters during stroke'. By RicHard-59 - Own work, based on File:Activated NMDAR.PNG, CC BY-SA 3.0, https://commons.wikimedia.o

cause the neuron to die, a process known as **apoptosis**.

Medical researchers have been striving for decades to prevent brain cell death with different **neuroprotective** drugs and blocking some of the abnormal processes described earlier. However, disappointingly, these extensive research efforts have failed to find a single effective

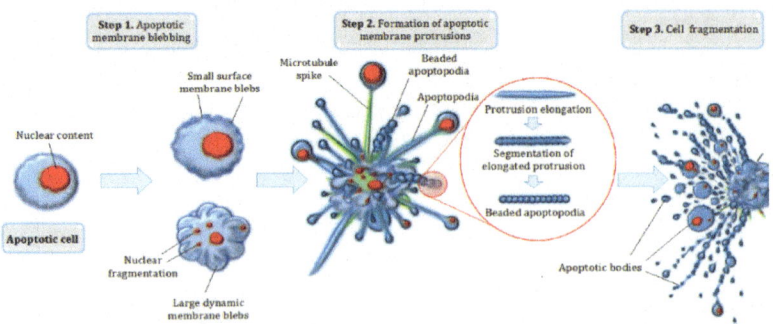
'Apoptotic cell disassembly'. By Aaron Smith, Michael AF Parkes, Georgia K Atkin-Smith, Rochelle Tixeira, Ivan KH Poon / CC BY (https://creativecommons.org/licenses/by/4.0)

neuroprotective treatment that is actually effective in humans.

The things that have been found to be successful actually seem rather simple in comparison to the elegant theories behind neuroprotective drugs. Simply cooling the body or brain tissue appears to prevent further damage. This approach, known as **therapeutic hypothermia**, has been employed to treat brain injury in patients who have suffered a complete cardiac arrest. So far though, hypothermia has not been found to be practical for treatment of stroke. Restoring blood circulation to the brain arteries has proven to be the only truly effective method of treating acute ischemic stroke. The use of TPA/alteplase and the newer treatment of thrombectomy/clot retrieval have dramatically altered the outlook for stroke victims.

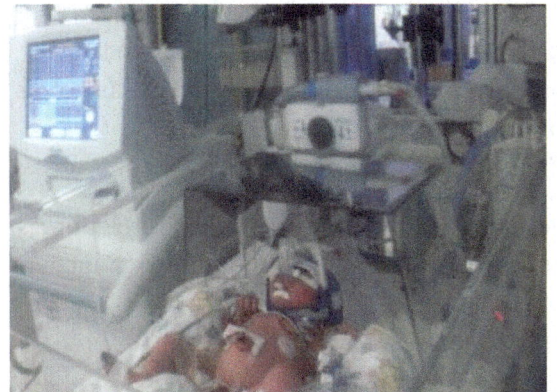

'Therapeutic hypothermia with head cooling device used for newborn with hypoxic brain injury'. By Enuice Diaz. Flickr. CC BY 2.0.

In order to understand the reason due to which restoring blood circulation aids the ischemic brain, we must remember why blood flow was affected in the first place. As we learned in chapter 1, blood flow can be blocked by several different processes such as lacunar infarcts or arterial dissections and not necessarily due to a clot or plug. However, the majority of strokes are caused due to some type of clot or debris plugging the pathway or lumen of the artery. Most of these clots were formed on the surface of the arteries, known as atherosclerotic arteries. Other clots form within the heart due to atrial fibrillation. The clots will detach and float downstream into smaller and smaller arteries until the clot becomes stuck. Blood is like a living tissue. It is full of enzymes and molecules and different cells that fight disease and cancer, carry oxygen to tissue and take away waste products. At the same time, blood is also full of components for creating clots as well as dissolving clots.

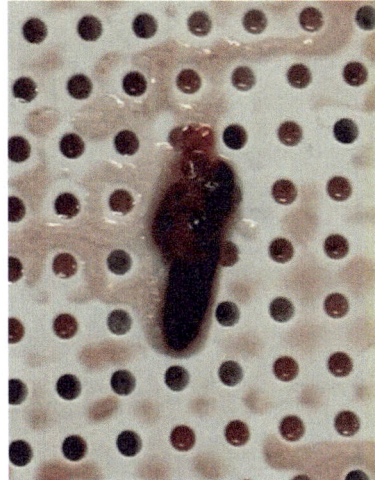 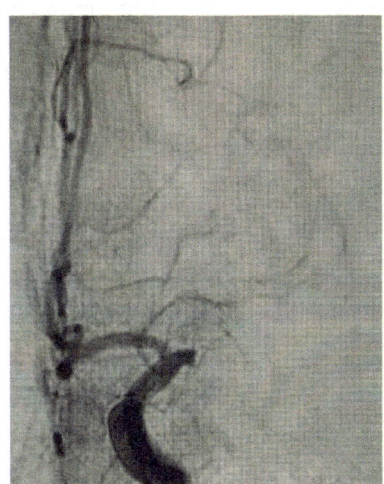 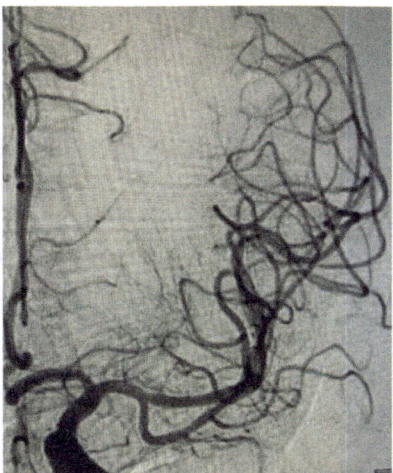

Clot removed from middle cerebral artery. Cerebral angiogram shows occlusion of the MCA and complete restoration of blood flow after successful thrombectomy. Courtesy Ben English, MD. St. Charles Medical Center.

Normal clot formation or **coagulation** occurs to prevent internal bleeding due to minor diseases or external bleeding due to minor trauma. The process of coagulation is extremely complex but basically

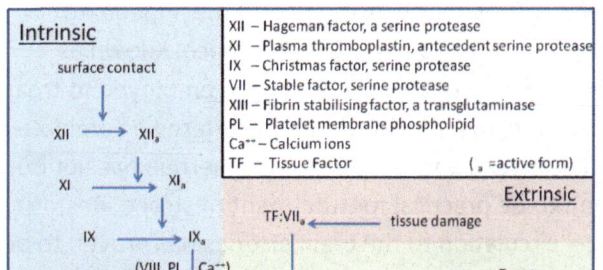

'Classical blood coagulation pathways'. By Dr Graham Beards. https://commons.wikimedia.org/w/index.php?curid=1909...

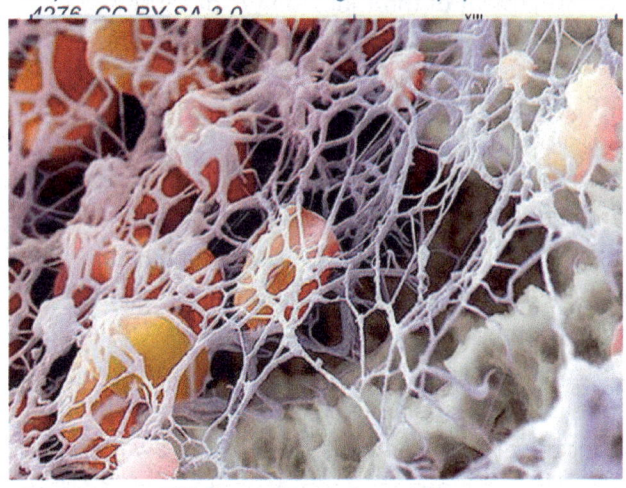

'Platelets and fibrin net formation within a thrombus'. https://beyondthedish.wordpress.com/category/stem-cell-eye-treatments/ CC BY-NC-ND 3.0.

involves three complicated interacting systems. These include molecules on the surface of the inner lining or endothelium of arteries, small blood cells designed for clot formation known as **platelets**, and the creation of molecular nets of **fibrin**, created from a circulating protein, **fibrinogen**.

Several drugs, referred to as anti-platelet drugs, currently available, inhibit the clotting function of platelets. These include aspirin and **clopidogrel** (Plavix). Moreover, weaker anti-platelet drugs such as **dipyridamole** or **cilostazol** (Pletal) can be combined with aspirin to achieve a more robust anti-clotting effect.

Another group of drugs, referred to as anticoagulant drugs, inhibit the creation of fibrin nets. These drugs work through several different molecular mechanisms and include intravenous, rapid acting drugs such as **heparin** or slower acting oral anticoagulants such as **warfarin** (Coumadin) as well as newer oral agents such as **apixaban** (Eliquis), **rivaroxaban** (Xarelto) and **dabigatran** (Pradaxa). These drugs are highly potent and carry the risk of excessive bleeding.

However, the process of coagulation must be regulated by the body or it could lead to clotting of all blood immediately. Therefore, thrombus formation is carefully balanced by the counter process of fibrinolysis, in which opposing enzymes digest clots. **Fibrinolysis** is largely controlled by a protein called **plasmin** formed from another protein known as **plasminogen.** TPA or alteplase functions by activating plasminogen and converting it into plasmin. TPA stands for tissue plasminogen activator.

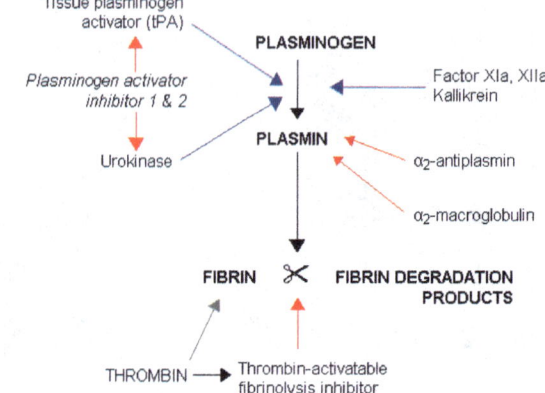

'Fibrinolysis'. By Jfdwolff at en.wikipedia. CC BY-SA 3.0.

Presently, only three drugs have found a role in the current immediate treatment of acute stroke. These are aspirin, heparin and TPA/alteplase. Multiple studies have demonstrated that treatment with aspirin within 48 hours of stroke onset is associated with reduced disability. This result is modest, but we still administer aspirin routinely to all stroke patients unless they are receiving TPA. However, note that we do not recommend administering aspirin to stroke victims before reaching the hospital. This is because some patients who appear to be having an ischemic stroke will turn out to have suffered a brain hemorrhage which might worsen due to aspirin. Heparin has only been studied once, years ago, for effectiveness in acute stroke. At that time, it proved to have no positive impact on the outcome and increased the risk of bleeding complications.

However, a new role for Heparin has now been found in the treatment of acute stroke in certain situations. Since CT angiography has enabled us to actually see clots, we can now observe that occasionally a clot will stick to an artery wall without completely occluding it. This situation known as non-occlusive clot can be found in a patient who showed TIA symptoms but is still in danger of completely occluding the artery and suffering a major stroke. These patients can be treated with intravenous heparin for several days to prevent the clot from growing and allowing it to stabilize then dissolving by the body's natural process of fibrinolysis.

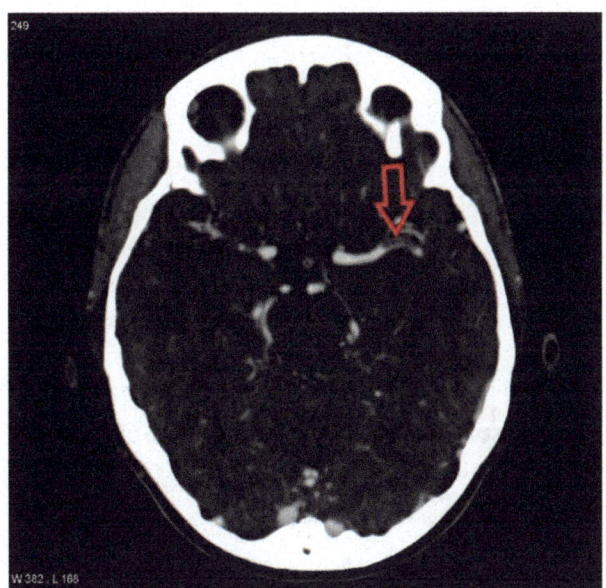

'Nonocclusive thrombus in the middle cerebral artery'. Case courtesy of Assoc Prof Frank Gaillard, <a href="https://radiopaedia.org/">Radiopaedia.org</a>. From the case <a href="https://radiopaedia.org/cases/4587">rID: 4587</a>

The treatment of stroke was revolutionized in 1995 when successful treatment with TPA or tissue plasminogen activator, also called alteplase, was first reported in the New England Journal of Medicine.[5] Even back in the 1930s, researchers were discovering enzymes such as streptokinase or urokinase which would activate plasmin, the enzyme that dissolves acute clots. Beginning in the 1960s, physicians were learning how to use these drugs to treat heart attacks due to coronary artery thrombosis. Eventually, urokinase was used in small trials for stroke. The tissue plasminogen activator was discovered in 1979 and has proved to be even more effective than urokinase for clot lysis and found to be safer with regard to hemorrhagic complications.

Several commercial brands of TPA are available; the one that is FDA approved for stroke is **alteplase** (Activase). Another type of TPA, **tenecteplase**, may actually prove to be more successful and could possibly replace alteplase in the future.[6]

---

[5] Tissue Plasminogen Activator for Acute Ischemic Stroke
N Engl J Med 1995; 333:1581–1588
The National Institute of Neurological Disorders and Stroke rt-PA Stroke Study Group
[6] Tenecteplase versus Alteplase before Thrombectomy for Ischemic Stroke

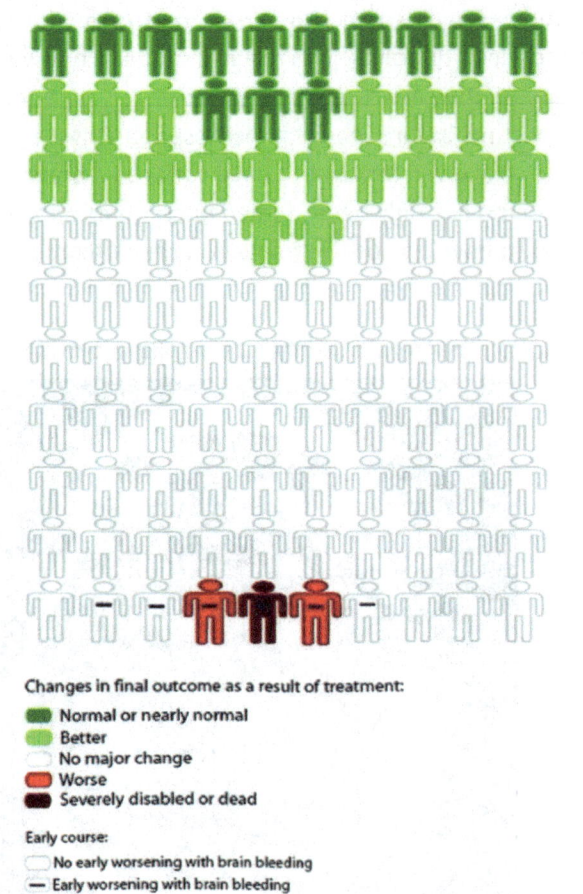

'Visual decision aid to help patients and families assess benefits and risks of thrombolytic therapy within the first 3 hours of onset'.
Courtesy of UCLA Stroke Center. Image publicly available under a Creative Commons Use with Attribution license.

Research and clinical experience have repeatedly demonstrated that TPA is most effective if administered quickly after the onset of stroke. Otherwise, it becomes less effective for dissolving the clot. The clot becomes firmer with each passing minute. Moreover, as the artery and brain die, lysis of the clot could allow blood flow to reenter a dead artery, which could lead to a rupture resulting in a severe or fatal brain hemorrhage. The original study showed that TPA could be given with relative safety up to three hours after the onset of stroke and later studies have shown this can be extended to 4.5 hours in many cases. Beyond that, the risk of hemorrhage clearly outweighs any potential benefit. The original studies revealed that an additional 31% of stroke victims who are given TPA make a good recovery as compared to those who do not receive the treatment.

However, 6.4% of patients who are given TPA may develop hemorrhage in brain tissue. The hemorrhage can sometimes be severe or even fatal but more commonly does not affect the outcome. Patients who develop hemorrhages are more likely to be older, have larger strokes or have suffered a longer delay before receiving

---

N Engl J Med 2018; 378:1573–1582
Bruce CV Campbell, Ph.D., Peter J Mitchell, M.Med., Leonid Churilov, Ph.D., Nawaf Yassi, Ph.D., Timothy J Kleinig, Ph.D., Richard J Dowling, M.B., B.S., Bernard Yan, M.B., B.S., Steven J Bush, M.B., B.S., Helen M Dewey, M.D., Vincent Thijs, M.D., Rebecca Scroop, M.B., B.S., Marion Simpson, M.B., B.S., et al., for the EXTEND-IA TNK Investigators

treatment.

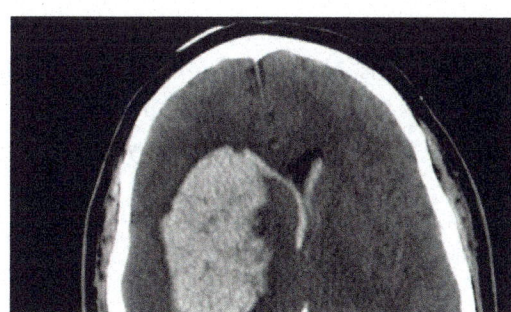
'TPA related cerebral hemorrhage'. Case courtesy of Dr Chris O'Donnell, <a href="https://radiopaedia.org/">Radiopaedia.org</a>. From the case <a href="https://radiopaedia.org/cases/19776">rID: 19776</a>

All doctors feel concerned that they may accidentally treat a patient with TPA who actually turns out to have a stroke. This can occur in certain neurological conditions, such as seizures or complicated migraines, which can show similar symptoms. These other conditions are referred to as **stroke mimics**. Fortunately, patients with stroke mimics tend to be the least likely to experience hemorrhage from TPA.

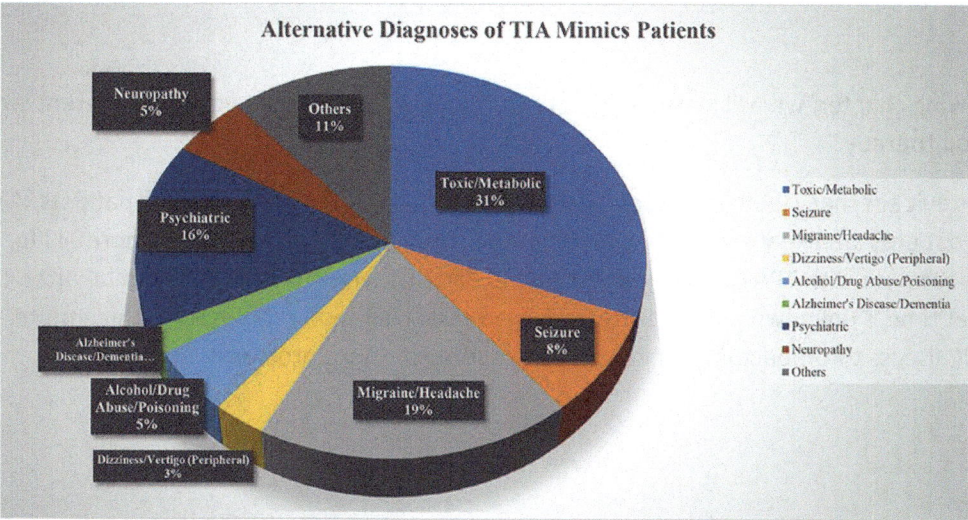
'Stroke mimics'. frontiersin.org/articles/10.3389/fneur.2019.00294/full. CC BY 4.0.

Another limitation is that TPA is most effective on smaller clots. Clots that have been present for longer periods, are longer (> 8 mm) or occlude larger vessels such as the internal carotid artery are less likely to respond to TPA.

Therefore, multiple steps need to take place before a patient can be treated with TPA. The patient needs to reach the hospital fast, then be examined by a physician trained in stroke care. Thereafter, alternative diagnoses have to be ruled out by a brain CT scan. There are multiple reasons due to which patients can be excluded from TPA treatment based on other medical problems. The AHA lists these contraindications in its guidelines. The exclusions include the patient taking an anticoagulant medication, recent major surgery, recent gastrointestinal bleeding, and pregnancy among numerous other reasons. The primary exclusion factor is time. If the time of stroke onset is unknown or if the symptoms have been present for more than 4.5 hours, TPA is almost never provided. This concept is referred to as **time-based therapy**.

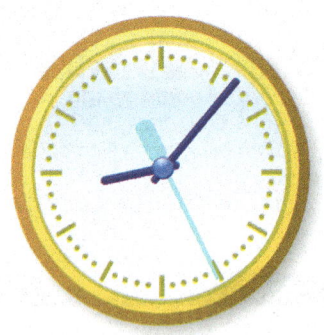

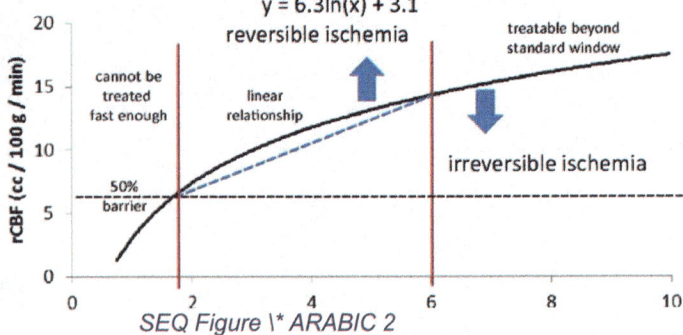

By Tkgd2007. Wikimedia Commons. CC0 1.0.

'Time to infarction after MCA occlusion'. Al-Ali F, Elias JJ and Filipkowski DE (2015) Acute ischemic stroke treatment, part 2: Treatment "Roles of capillary index score, revascularization and time". Front. Neurol. 6:117. doi: 10.3389/fneur.2015.00117. CC BY 4.0.

In the following chapter, we will learn more about time-based therapy as well as a different strategy, **image-based therapy**.

Overall, it is evident that TPA has a strong positive effect on the outcome of stroke patients. A greater number of patients are likely to be able to walk out of the hospital and return to a normal life, but certainly, treatment with TPA cannot help everyone. Patients who reached the hospital after 4.5 hours, whose onset time is unknown or who suffered large vessel occlusion require something more. The next chapter will discuss thrombectomy which addresses some of these problems.

Chapter 5. Interventional and Surgical Therapies for Acute Stroke

In the previous chapter, we reviewed the basic principles of thrombosis as a major cause for stroke. We also reviewed the role of different anti-thrombotic drugs, particularly TPA, in treating acute stroke. The widespread utilization of TPA for acute stroke was a major breakthrough in the 1990s and continues to be a highly crucial treatment for patients who present with stroke symptoms within 4.5 hours. However, several patients fail to meet this requirement for treatment with TPA or are unable to communicate their symptoms onset time. For these patients, the risk of TPA causing intracranial hemorrhage is extremely high. Qualification for TPA is firmly based on knowing the time of onset of symptoms, referred to as "**last seen normal**", and treatment within the window of safety. This is known as **time-based therapy**. We are also aware that extremely large clots, particularly clots within large vessels such as the internal carotid artery or middle cerebral artery, do not respond well to TPA.

As it turns out, simply removing the thrombus that is plugging the flow through the critical artery is the most effective treatment for the most severe strokes. However, removing the clot is a delicate procedure that needs to be performed by a neurosurgeon, neurologist or interventional radiologist with the requisite training and experience to perform this treatment. The first challenge is for emergency responders to recognize which patient with stroke symptoms would qualify for clot retrieval, the process also referred to as **thrombectomy**.

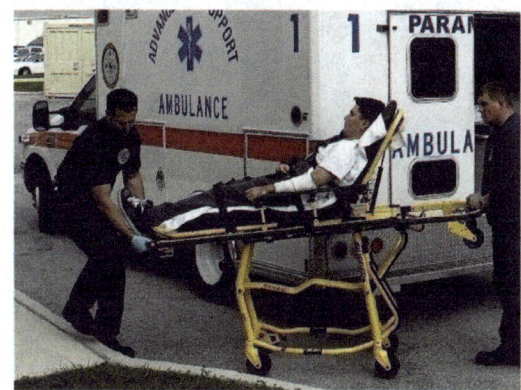

'Paramedics performing drill'. Public Domain.

In Chapter 3, we reviewed several scoring systems employed by EMS responders. In Central Oregon, it is **C-STAT**. This very quick and easy to perform scoring system is based on a simple examination. Patients who are **C-STAT positive**, also referred to as **LVO stroke patients**, meaning those with large vessel occlusion, need to be transported to a hospital where thrombectomy can be performed as early as possible. This may require the patient to be transported directly to Bend, bypassing closer hospitals that might offer TPA but cannot provide thrombectomy. In the near future, all EMS systems in Central Oregon will employ the same triage system which will encourage rapid transport of LVO patients directly to Bend. Due to the challenges presented by such a large geographical area, the use of air ambulance services is encouraged as well. SAO and the St. Charles Stroke Program both steer all families to purchase inexpensive air ambulance insurance for citizens in Central Oregon.

CINCINNATI STROKE TRIAGE ASSESSMENT TOOL - C-STAT		
	Points	Definition
GAZE		Unable to look in certain direction with both eyes.
Absent (Normal)	0	
Present (Abnormal)	2	
ARM WEAKNESS		Cannot hold up arm(s) for 10 seconds.
Absent (Normal)	0	
Present (Abnormal)	1	
LEVEL OF CONCSIOUSNESS		Incorrectly answers at least one of two LOC questions AND does not follow at least one of two commands.
Absent (Normal)	0	LOC Questions-What month is it? How old are you?
Present (Abnormal)	1	LOC Commands-Open your eyes. Make a fist.
C-STAT positive is defined as a score of ≥ 2		

Courtesy East Cascades EMS Council.

In 2018, two articles published in the New England Journal of Medicine described thrombectomy for patients with stroke symptoms occurring even up to 24 hours earlier, based on the findings of imaging techniques rather than time alone. These were the **DAWN Study** and **DEFUSE-3 Study**.[7][8] The DAWN Study revealed that patients treated with thrombectomy had a 49% chance of recovery to functional independence compared to 13% for patients who did not receive thrombectomy. These studies created a revolution in the care of patients with severe strokes. A different principle for deciding whether a patient is a candidate for thrombectomy entails using imaging procedures. Rather than using strict time guidelines, the decision is based on the imaging findings, known as **image-based therapy**. There are several remarkable imaging techniques that allow physicians to actually see how much brain tissue has died and how much is still surviving. The dead part is referred to as the **core infarct**. This is brain tissue that cannot be revived and could also be a source of hemorrhage if the arterial circulation to the core was reopened. Surrounding the core is an area that has diminished blood flow but the tissue is barely surviving. This is referred to as the **ischemic penumbra.** The term ischemic means loss of blood flow. Penumbra refers to a partial shadow such as that witnessed in a partial solar eclipse. The brain tissue inside the penumbra area may survive longer because it lies at the edge of the area supplied by the blocked artery. Thus, the penumbra survives longer because it may be receiving a small amount of blood from neighboring arteries. This is called **collateral blood flow**. As time passes, collateral blood flow will become inadequate, causing tissue within the penumbra to eventually die and form a part of the core.

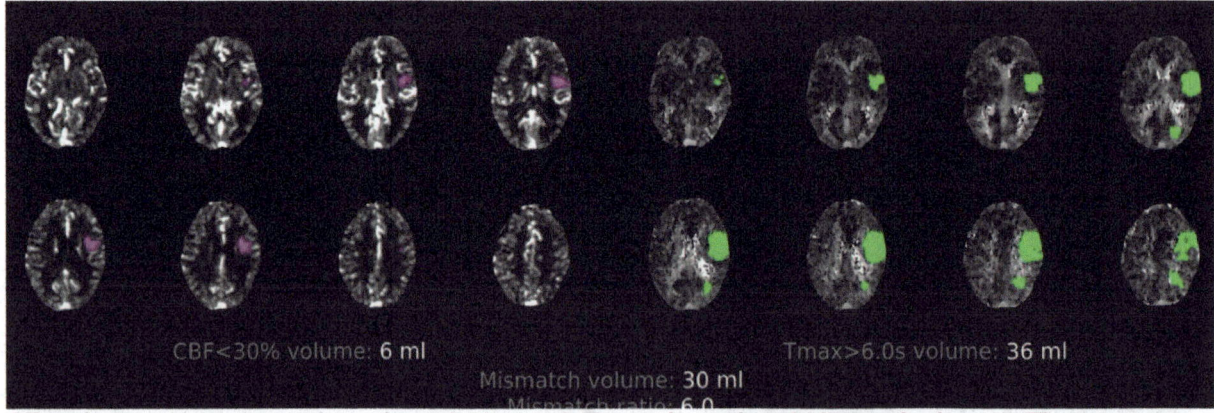

CT prefusion study of a stroke patient who has embolic stroke to the middle cerebral artery. The green area represents the ischemic penumbra. Pink is the ischemic core. The relatively greater proportion of penumbra vs core made this patiient a candidate for thrombectomy. This is known as imaged based therapy. Courtesy Steve Goins, MD.

---

[7] DAWN Study
Thrombectomy 6 to 24 Hours after Stroke with a Mismatch between Deficit and Infarct
N Engl J Med 2018; 378:11-21
Raul G. Nogueira, M.D., Ashutosh P. Jadhav, M.D., Ph.D., Diogo C. Haussen, M.D., Alain Bonafe, M.D., Ronald F. Budzik, M.D., Parita Bhuva, M.D., Dileep R. Yavagal, M.D., Marc Ribo, M.D., Christophe Cognard, M.D., Ricardo A. Hanel, M.D., Cathy A. Sila, M.D., Ameer E. Hassan, D.O., et al., for the DAWN Trial Investigators

[8] DEFUSE 3 Study
Thrombectomy for Stroke at 6 to 16 Hours with Selection by Perfusion Imaging
N Engl J Med 2018; 378:708–718
Gregory W Albers, M.D., Michael P Marks, M.D., Stephanie Kemp, B.S., Soren Christensen, Ph.D., Jenny P Tsai, M.D., Santiago Ortega-Gutierrez, M.D., Ryan A McTaggart, M.D., Michel T Torbey, M.D., May Kim-Tenser, M.D., Thabele Leslie-Mazwi, M.D., Amrou Sarraj, M.D., Scott E Kasner, M.D., et al., for the DEFUSE 3 Investigators

Of course, it is important to reestablish flow to the penumbra before the core grows to the point that hemorrhage risk becomes excessively high or treatment becomes futile.

CT perfusion, or **CTP**, is a technique in which the CT computer is used to analyze the flow of contrast injected into the bloodstream while a CT of the brain is performed at the same time. Using complicated computer programs, maps of the penumbra and core can be generated within a few minutes. Typically, CTP is performed at the same time a brain CT and CTA are conducted. However, CTP is extremely expensive, and this test is currently only available in Bend, where it is routinely performed for patients whose stroke symptoms have been present for more than six hours but less than 24 hours. Moreover, it is performed for patients who wake up with stroke symptoms. This condition is referred to as **wake-up stroke.** Until recently, there was no safe treatment available for patients with wake-up stroke even though nearly 1/3rd of all strokes occur during sleep.

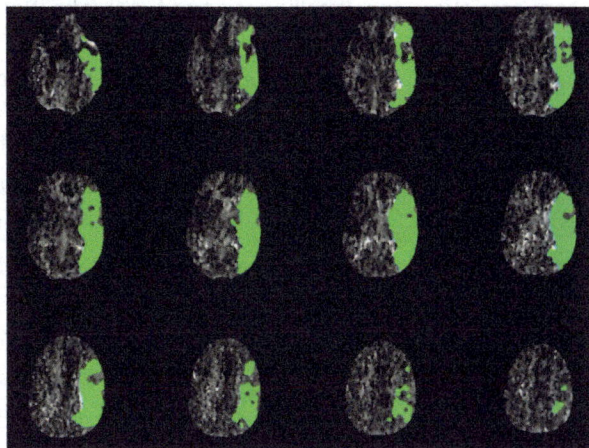
Another CTP demonstarting a large penumbra and no core in a patient who developed stroke symptoms 9 hours earlier. He probably received very good collateral flow and ultimately did well after thrombectomy. Courtesy Steve Goins, MD.

Brain MRI can also provide maps of the penumbra and core; however, the time required for performing an MRI is so long that it is usually considered impractical for an acute stroke situation.

Another interesting imaging method in this regard is a routine non-contrast brain CT and a score known as **ASPECTS**. ASPECTS (Alberta Stroke Program Early CT score) is a method in which a trained physician can kind of map out areas of core infarct with the naked eye or the assistance of a computer program. This is not nearly as reliable as a CTP, but it can be used as a screening tool to decide which patients would benefit by air ambulance transport from outlying hospitals to Bend. It is likely that ASPECTS will be increasingly utilized in Central Oregon hospitals to determine whether the patient should be transferred to Bend or not.

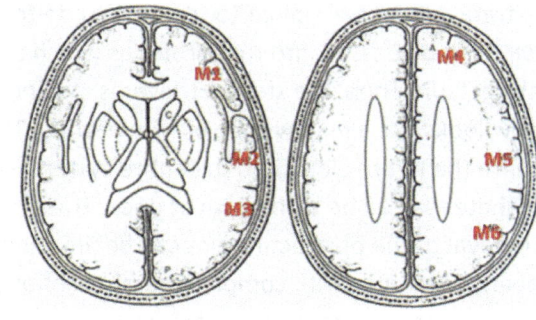
'Cerebral regions by ASPECTS'. commons.wikimedia.org/wiki/File:Cerebral_regions _by_ASPECTS.png. CC BY 4.0.

The development of thrombectomy treatments for stroke has only been realized in recent years but the concept has been around since the late 1920s. Physicians gradually learned how to use catheters inserted into peripheral arteries to access diseased or occluded arteries in other parts of the body. At first, this approach was merely used for peripheral vascular disease affecting arterial circulation of limbs. Later on, it was applied to cardiology for treatment of cardiac arrest. By the 1980s, attempts to use it for stroke had been made, but the initial technology was not reliable. Different catheter devices have been developed over time and efforts have been made to find a better method to snare the obstructing clot. Corkscrew devices were replaced by an extendable coiling system known as the MERCI device. By the late 1980s, doctors were experimenting with **stent retrievers**, devices that extrude from the tip of the catheter and then expand into a tiny wire net which can encompass the clot. The clot is then dragged out along with the catheter. Stent retrievers specifically designed for stroke were thereafter developed and have become the primary device for thrombectomy. Stent retrievers are faster and significantly more reliable than older systems and are 90% effective in removing clots.[9] [10]

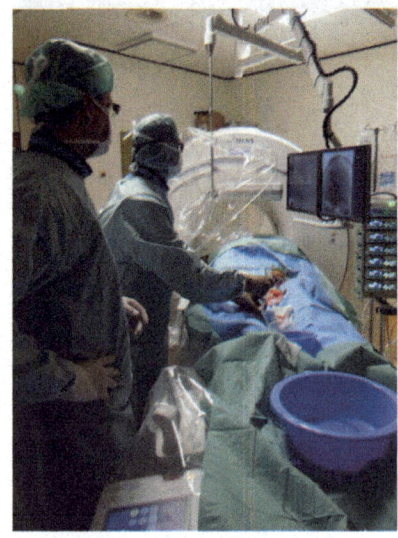

'Mechanical thrombectomy for stroke'.
https://jnis.bmj.com/content/8/6/621.
CC BY-NC 4.0.

Once a patient has been found to have a large vessel occlusion stroke, confirmed by CTA and possibly CT perfusion, they may still receive TPA if time allows. But the primary focus at this point becomes getting the patient to the special procedure suite in the radiology department as soon as possible. There, the interventional neurosurgeon or radiologist will perform a puncture in the patient's groin and introduce a catheter into the femoral artery. This very narrow but long catheter contains an internal wire guide that can be removed. Using the wire guide and by observing the passage of the catheter by X-ray, the physician can gradually guide the catheter tip up through the aorta and then carefully guide it further until it goes up the chosen right or left carotid artery or in some cases one of the vertebral arteries. The catheter can eventually be guided into arteries inside the skull, usually one of the middle cerebral arteries or possibly the basilar artery where the thrombus has lodged. Once the catheter tip is next to the clot, the doctor will remove the wire guide, leaving the catheter in place. Subsequently, a different wire system is introduced into the catheter. The stent retriever is now at the tip of the new wire. Before the stent retriever is expanded, it is extremely narrow, similar to the wire guide that it replaced. This new wire can be passed into the thrombus which at this point is still soft like gelatin. Then, the stent retriever is expanded. The expanded stent now looks like a hollow tube of wire netting. This stent can effectively snare the entire clot. Then the entire system, stent retriever, clot and catheter can all be withdrawn at once. The effect of this sudden removal of the obstructing clot can be amazing. Patients who are nearly comatose with complete paralysis of one side may suddenly wake up and start moving all limbs!

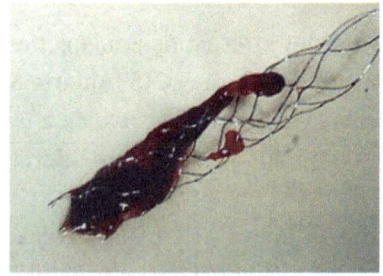

'Stent retriever used successfully'.
https://pn.bmj.com/content/17/4/252

---

[9] Stent-Retriever Thrombectomy after Intravenous t-PA vs. t-PA Alone in Stroke
N Engl J Med 2015; 372:2285–2295
Jeffrey L Saver, M.D., Mayank Goyal, M.D., Alain Bonafe, M.D., Hans-Christoph Diener, M.D., Ph.D., Elad I Levy, M.D., Vitor M Pereira, M.D., Gregory W Albers, M.D., Christophe Cognard, M.D., David J Cohen, M.D., Werner Hacke, M.D., Ph.D., Olav Jansen, M.D., Ph.D., Tudor G Jovin, M.D., et al., for the SWIFT PRIME Investigators

[10] Randomized Assessment of Rapid Endovascular Treatment of Ischemic Stroke
N Engl J Med 2015; 372:1019–1030
Mayank Goyal, M.D., Andrew M. Demchuk, M.D., Bijoy K Menon, M.D., Muneer Eesa, M.D., Jeremy L Rempel, M.D., John Thornton, M.D., Daniel Roy, M.D., Tudor G Jovin, M.D., Robert A Willinsky, M.D., Biggya L Sapkota, M.B., B.S., Dar Dowlatshahi, M.D., Ph.D., Donald F Frei, M.D., et al., for the ESCAPE Trial Investigators

Patients who have undergone thrombectomy or treatment TPA will then spend the next 24 hours in the intensive care unit. They are monitored continuously with hourly nursing evaluations. Their blood pressure is carefully regulated for the particular situation. Occasionally, patients who have suffered a severe stroke but were then treated with TPA and thrombectomy fully recover and are discharge directly from the ICU.

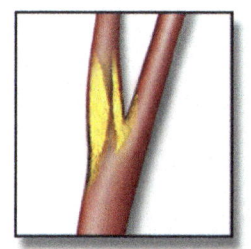

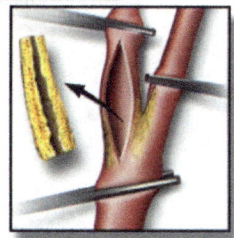

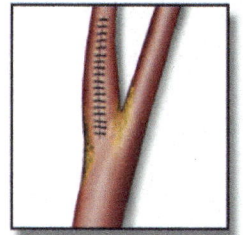

'Carotid endarterectomy'.
https://en.wikiversity.org/wiki/WikiJournal_of_Medicine/Medical_gallery_of_Blausen_Medical_2014. CC BY 3.0.

Interventional neurosurgeons also perform a variety of other endovascular procedures for other situations. This may include procedures to close cerebral aneurysms or to place stents within critically narrowed brain arteries before a stroke occurs. There are also several procedures for opening critically narrowed internal carotid arteries. The oldest and perhaps most reliable procedure is **carotid endarterectomy**,[11] in which the surgeon cuts open the narrowed artery and shells out the diseased internal lining or intima of the artery before sewing the artery close again. Carotid arteries that are narrowed beyond 70% pose a high risk for eventually causing stroke and are often treated with carotid endartectomy. A more recent development is **carotid stenting**, which allows avoiding an open surgery and the diseased carotid artery is opened with an expandable stent, which is larger and much stiffer than the small stent retrievers used for stroke. An even more recent variation of carotid stenting is referred to as **TCAR (transcarotid artery revascularization)**. This is an innovative carotid procedure in which blood flow to the brain is actually reversed while a stent is placed in the diseased carotid artery. This reversal of blood flow prevents atherosclerotic debris, dislodged by the stent placement, from flowing up into the smaller arteries of the brain. Therefore, the risk of a stroke complication is substantially reduced.

'Carotid stenting'. Public Domain.

In this and the previous chapter, we reviewed a fairly detailed description of the current prominent treatments for acute stroke. In real life, every patient's situation is unique, often accompanied by other medical complications. Successful treatment depends on rapid recognition of stroke symptoms, accurate triage and transport by EMS providers and rapid, parallel communication between the different

---

[11] Beneficial Effect of Carotid Endarterectomy in Symptomatic Patients with High-Grade Carotid Stenosis
N Engl J Med 1991; 325:445–453
North American Symptomatic Carotid Endarterectomy Trial Collaborators

members of the hospital stroke team. The stroke team comprises doctors, nurses, technicians, communication operators and numerous other supporting members. The only way that this complex system can work is if everyone involved knows their job precisely and strives to communicate with other team members efficiently. Every minute of delay costs nearly 2 million brain cells and everyone should keep this consequence in mind. A few minutes of delay here or there could make the difference whether between a life of disability and complete recovery.

Chapter 6. Secondary Prevention of Stroke

Unfortunately, people who have survived a stroke face significant risk of recurrence. The **Oxfordshire Community Stroke Project** published in 1994 revealed that stroke survivors face 15 times greater risk of a recurrent stroke than the general population. The risk of stroke during the first year was 13% and the five-year risk was 30%.[12] However, this risk is not distributed equally among all stroke survivors. Some of the younger stroke patients actually have a very slight risk of recurrence while some have a very high risk due to multiple risk factors that accumulate with age and lifestyle. Thus, the risk can be stratified based on an individual's risk factors. All patients who survive stroke need to have a thorough evaluation to identify their modifiable and unmodifiable risk factors.

Similarly, patients who have had a TIA also need to have careful evaluation of their modifiable and unmodifiable risk factors. After a TIA, the annual stroke risk is 3%–4% overall, but this is particularly high during the first 24 hours and a month after the TIA. Conversely, 12–30%of patients who have stroke have had a preceding TIA. A quarter of these TIAs occurred immediately prior to the stroke. Again, the risk for a particular individual can be stratified based on different risk factors. Immediate intervention post a TIA may reduce the stroke risk by 80%.

This chapter will focus on two important medical interventions, occlusive atherosclerotic large vessel disease and recognition and treatment of atrial fibrillation. Subsequently, important modifiable risk factors will also be reviewed.

The single most important issue to resolve in the initial evaluation of TIA and ischemic stroke is whether or not there is an obstructive lesion in a larger artery to the affected brain territory. Non-invasive options for evaluation of large vessel occlusive disease include magnetic resonance angiography (MRA), computed tomography angiography (CTA), carotid duplex ultrasonography (CDUS) and transcranial Doppler ultrasonography (TCD). The choice among these depends upon local availability and expertise as well as individual patient characteristics and preferences.

Recognition of atherosclerotic narrowing of the internal carotid artery in the neck as a cause for stroke was suspected even in the early 1900s. In the 1950s, the eminent stroke neurologist C. Miller Fisher promoted understanding of carotid artery disease as a major cause of stroke. He wrote: "unexplained cerebral embolism may arise from thrombotic material lying in the carotid sinus", and "it is even conceivable that someday, vascular surgery will find a way to bypass the occluded portion of the artery during the period of ominous fleeting symptoms".

C. Miller Fisher was correct. High-grade carotid narrowing or stenosis proved to be a major cause of stroke. The phenomenon was only occasionally caused due to decreased blood flow across the narrowed segment. The primary problem was that the narrowing was a result of atherosclerosis, deposition of cholesterol within the middle layer or media of the artery wall. This happened because there is a peculiar pattern of turbulence of blood flow that occurs at this location where the common carotid artery branches into the internal and external carotid arteries.

---

[12] Long-term risk of recurrent stroke after a first-ever stroke. The Oxfordshire Community Stroke Project.
J Burn, M Dennis, J Bamford, P Sandercock, D Wade, and C Warlow
Originally published 1 Feb 1994 https://doi.org/10.1161/01.STR.25.2.333Stroke. 1994;25:333–337

As we learned in Chapter 1, the cholesterol accumulation gradually overwhelms the ability of macrophages to contain it. Eventually, the cholesterol plaque becomes inflamed and causes deterioration of the inner lining or intima. The intima then gets ulcerated and this is where clots form. The clots or thrombus subsequently detach and travel with blood to arteries in the brain until they become lodged in smaller but critical arteries. Paradoxically, if an internal carotid artery gradually closes completely, it actually forms a safer situation since clots are no longer forming.

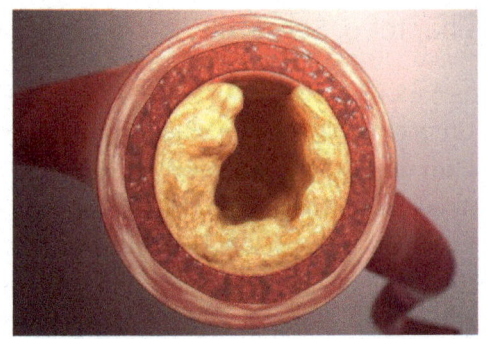

'Clogged artery'. Scientific Animations, Girish Khera / CC BY-SA

Over the following decade, carotid endarterectomy, a method of opening the artery and removing the diseased inner layer or atherosclerotic intima became a commonly performed procedure. Unfortunately, awareness about the significance of carotid disease was not accompanied by enhancement in surgical technique. Surgery proved to be risky and could result in stroke or even death during these early years.

National Heart Lung and Blood Insitute (NIH) / Public domain

In 1991, the results of the **North American Symptomatic Carotid Endarterectomy Trial** were published.[13] This study clarified the risk concurrent with different degrees of carotid stenosis for both symptomatic and asymptomatic patients. **NASCET** demonstrated a highly beneficial effect of carotid endarterectomy in patients with angiographically confirmed high-grade carotid stenosis (70% to 99%).

---

[13] Beneficial Effect of Carotid Endarterectomy in Symptomatic Patients with High-Grade Carotid Stenosis
N Engl J Med 1991; 325:445–453
North American Symptomatic Carotid Endarterectomy Trial Collaborators

For patients with stenosis <70%, the study revealed modest benefit from carotid endarterectomy in selected patients with moderate degrees of stenosis (50% to 69%).

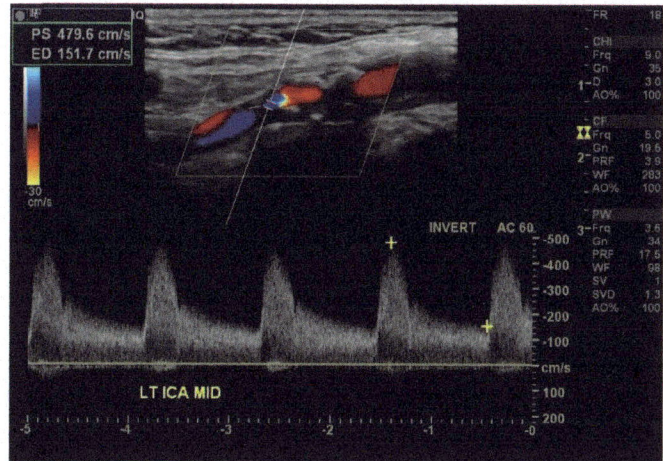

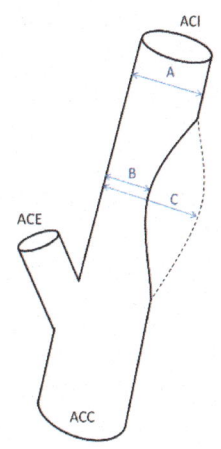

'Carotid Stenosis demonstrated by ultrasound'.

Mme Mim / CC BY-SA (https://creativecommons.org/licenses/by-sa/3.0)

'Diagram used for determining the grade of carotid stenosis according to NASCET'.

Today, the number of possible interventional options for carotid stenosis have increased. **Carotid stenting** is an alternative for high-risk patients instead of open surgery for carotid endarterectomy. More recently, **TCAR** or **Trans-Carotid Artery Revascularization** has been developed, which likely presents an even lower risk option compared to carotid stenting or endarterectomy.

Previously, we discussed the importance of atrial fibrillation as a cause for stroke. Atrial fibrillation, sometimes referred to as **"a-Fib"**, refers to abnormal rapid irregular beating of the left atrium or upper chamber of the heart. Left atrium is not a main pumping chamber; it rather pre-loads blood into the main pumping chamber or ventricle. These rapid contractions of the heart result in sluggish blood flow into the atrium. As the blood stagnates, it can form clots. These clots will dislodge and be pumped out by the heart and travel up to the arteries of the brain. There, the clot will become a plug and block blood flow causing a stroke. Atrial fibrillation becomes remarkably common as people get older. In America, 2.2 million people have a-fib. Several people can tolerate a- Fib, but the risk of atrial fibrillation causing stroke increases with age. By the age of 80, atrial fibrillation may become the cause of 1 in 4 strokes.

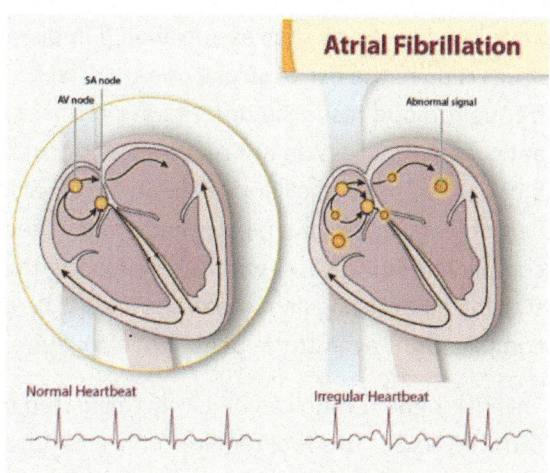

https://www.cdc.gov/heartdisease/images/atrial-fibrillation-medium.jpg

Atrial fibrillation is tricky. Many experience no symptoms and have no awareness that they are going in and out of atrial fibrillation. After one episode of atrial fibrillation, the likelihood of more episodes becomes 90%. Moreover, 90% of these episodes, even long episodes lasting up to 48 hours, are not recognized by the person.

Cardiac monitoring is an essential part of evaluation to exclude atrial fibrillation in the setting of embolic TIA or stroke. Cardiac rhythm monitoring with inpatient telemetry, Ziopatch study or Holter monitor are useful for patients without a clear cause for their TIA or stroke symptoms. With the advent of new, readily available technology, people can screen themselves using atrial fibrillation detecting apps on the Apple watch or using devices such as Kardia. However, whether the use of Apple watch actually reduces the risk of stroke has not yet been proven.

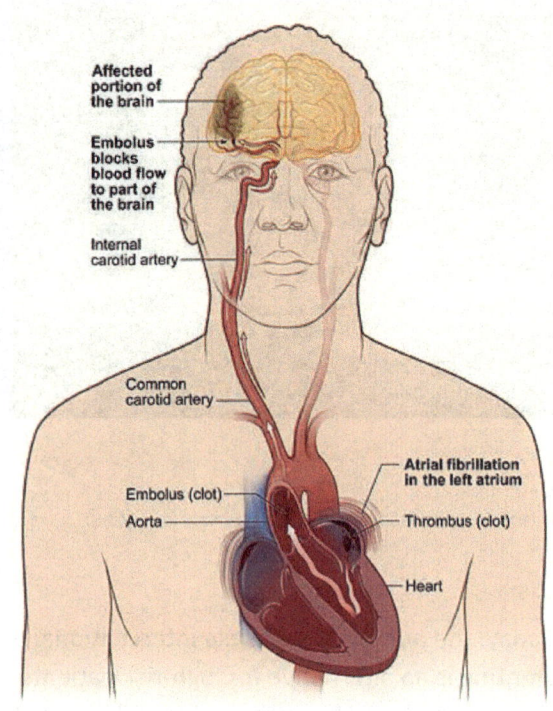

National Heart Lung and Blood Institute (NIH) / Public domain

While atrial fibrillation can often be difficult to detect, fortunately, effective treatment with anticoagulant medications is possible. Antiplatelet drugs such as aspirin or clopidigrel have not been shown to prevent atrial clotting or stroke. In contrast, anticoagulant drugs that work on thrombin and fibrin formation in clot development have been repeatedly demonstrated to be effective in reducing clot formation and stroke. Anticoagulant medications include warfarin (Coumadin) and newer, expensive direct acting anticoagulant drugs such as apixaban (Eliquis), rivaroxaban (Xarelto) and dabigatran (Pradaxa). These drugs reduce the risk of stroke due to atrial fibrillation by at least 75%. Warfarin therapy requires frequent blood testing in order to avoid the risk of making the excessively thin. The newer direct acting anticoagulant drugs do not require blood test monitoring and may be safer in terms of over thinning of blood. Nonetheless, all anticoagulant drugs also carry the risk of major bleeding complications including hemorrhage in the brain, gastrointestinal bleeding or even external bleeding. The risk of bleeding complications increases with age, mirroring the rising risk of stroke from atrial fibrillation. The choice of starting an anticoagulant medication must be made carefully, balancing the risks of hemorrhagic complications against the benefit of stroke prevention.

This risk-benefit ratio can be easily calculated for a person using statistically proven models such as **CHA2DS-VASc.** This tool requires only a minute of a doctor's time and estimates the risk-benefit based on the patient's age, gender and comorbidities including heart failure, hypertension, diabetes, history of previous stroke and vascular disease. **CHA2DS2-VASc** and its variations should be employed routinely when a person is discovered to have atrial fibrillation.

	CHA$_2$DS$_2$-VASc	
	Condition	Points
C	Congestive heart failure (or Left ventricular systolic dysfunction)	1
H	Hypertension: blood pressure consistently above 140/90 mmHg (or treated hypertension on medication)	1
A$_2$	Age ≥75 years	2
D	Diabetes Mellitus	1
S$_2$	Prior Stroke or TIA or thromboembolism	2
V	Vascular disease (e.g. peripheral artery disease, myocardial infarction, aortic plaque)	1
A	Age 65–74 years	1
Sc	Sex category (i.e. female sex)	1

Annual Stroke Risk		
CHA$_2$DS$_2$-VASc Score	Stroke Risk %	95% CI
0	0	-
1	1.3	-
2	2.2	-
3	3.2	-
4	4.0	-
5	6.7	-
6	9.8	-
7	9.6	-
8	12.5	-
9	15.2	-

'Prevention of stroke in patients with atrial fibrillation: current strategies and future directions'. Hohnloser, SH; Duray, GZ; Baber, U; Halperin, JL. European Heart Journal Supplements. British Medical Journal. (2008).10: H4–H10. doi:10.1093/eurheartj/sun029

All people, particularly those who have suffered a stroke or TIA, require counseling regarding the importance of major modifiable risk factors. The most common and important risk factors are:

- Hypertension
- Elevated cholesterol or other lipid disorders
- Tobacco use
- Diabetes
- Physical inactivity.

The impact of these five conditions clearly begins during adolescence. The **Pathobiological Determinants of Atherosclerosis in Youth (PDAY)** study was organized to document the natural history of atherosclerosis and determine the relation of cardiovascular risk factors to atherosclerosis in young subjects.[14] The PDAY study was a 10-year study involving 15 medical centers throughout the USA. Pathology laboratories in 15 medical centers collected coronary arteries, aortas and other tissues from over 3,000 subjects aged between 15 to 34 years who died of external causes between 1987 and 1994. This study revealed extensive atherosclerosis of the aorta to have 300% greater surface involvement in teens with multiple risk factors.

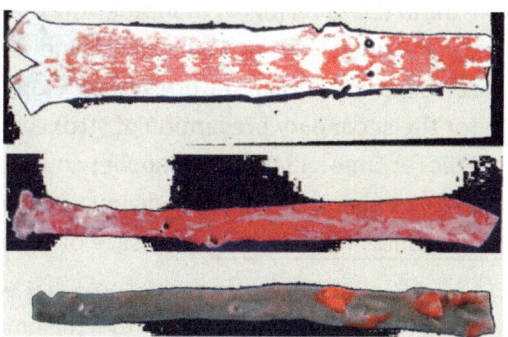

'Aortic specimens showing extensive plaquing. The PDAY Study: natural history, risk factors, and pathobiology. Pathobiological Determinants of Atherosclerosis in Youth'. Strong et al. Ann N Y Acad Sci 1997 Apr 15;811:226–235

[14] Pathobiological determinants of atherosclerosis in youth risk scores are associated with early and advanced atherosclerosis.
Pediatrics. 2006 Oct;118(4):1447–1455
McMahan CA1, Gidding SS, Malcom GT, Tracy RE, Strong JP, McGill HC Jr; Pathobiological Determinants of Atherosclerosis in Youth Research Group.

Further, multiple studies have analyzed autopsies of young US servicemen who died during the last several wars. Again, these clearly indicate that atherosclerosis begins at an early age.

Additional modifiable risk factors include:

- Atherosclerotic narrowing of other arteries such as the middle cerebral artery, subclavian artery, vertebral artery or basilar artery.

- A variety of heart conditions including patent foramen ovale, myocardial infarction with thrombus, cardiomyopathy, valvular heart disease, prosthetic heart valve.

- A wide spectrum of blood disorders including inherited coagulation disorders, antiphospholipid antibody syndrome, sickle cell disease and polycythemia.

- Drug use, particularly methamphetamine and cocaine.

- Sleep apnea.

Management of patients who have experienced TIA is complicated because of the numerous variables involved and emerging treatments. The most recent recommendations from the American Heart Association for TIA (2014)[15] include the following:

For patients with noncardioembolic ischemic stroke or TIA, the use of antiplatelet agents is recommended over anticoagulation to reduce the risk of recurrent stroke or other cardiovascular events.

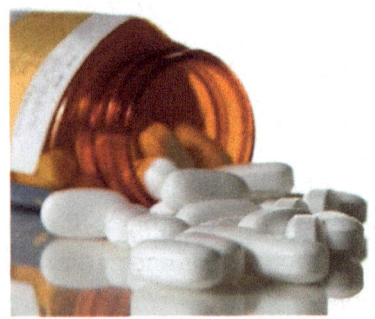

By Amanda Mills. pixnio.com. CC0

- Aspirin (50–3 25 mg/d) monotherapy or a combination of aspirin 25 mg and extended release dipyridamole 200 mg twice daily is indicated as the initial therapy after TIA or ischemic stroke for the prevention of future stroke. Clopidogrel 75 mg monotherapy is a reasonable alternative for the secondary prevention of stroke in place of aspirin or combination aspirin/dipyridamole. This recommendation also applies to patients who are allergic to aspirin. The selection of anti-platelet agents should be individualized on the basis of patient risk factor profiles, cost, tolerance, relative known efficacy of the agents and other clinical characteristics.

---

[15] Guidelines for the Prevention of Stroke in Patients With Stroke and Transient Ischemic Attack
A Guideline for Healthcare Professionals From the American Heart Association/American Stroke Association
Walter N Kernan, Bruce Ovbiagele, Henry R Black, Dawn M Bravata, Marc I Chimowitz, Michael D Ezekowitz, Margaret C Fang, Marc Fisher, Karen L Furie, Donald V Heck, S Claiborne (Clay) Johnston, Scott E Kasner, Steven J Kittner, Pamela H Mitchell, Michael W Rich, DeJuran Richardson, Lee H Schwamm, and John A Wilson
and on behalf of the American Heart Association Stroke Council, Council on Cardiovascular and Stroke Nursing, Council on Clinical Cardiology, and Council on Peripheral Vascular Disease
Stroke. 2014;45:2160–2236

- The combination of aspirin and clopidogrel can be considered for initiation within 24 hours of a minor stroke or TIA and then continued for 21 days.

- The combination of aspirin and clopidogrel is recommended for 90 days in situations where intracranial arterial stenosis is suspected.

Since atherosclerosis is a major cause of stroke and elevated lipids, mainly LDL cholesterol, a primary factor for atherosclerosis, it seems obvious why the treatment of elevated cholesterol has a significant impact on the risk of future stroke or TIA. Our blood cholesterol level is comprised by cholesterol that we consume, mainly through meat, but another substantial portion is produced by our liver and this cannot be significantly changed by diet modifications. The amount of liver produced cholesterol appears to increase as people become older. While cholesterol levels can be improved with diet changes and some medications, the use of a type of cholesterol lowering drug referred to as statins is usually recommended. Statins have more than one effect. They lower the amount of liver produced cholesterol while also lowering inflammation within atherosclerotic plaques. Since inflamed plaques are more likely to form clots, this effect significantly reduces clot formation. It has also been demonstrated that statins actually reduce the size of plaques over time.

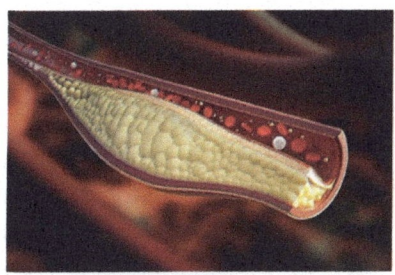
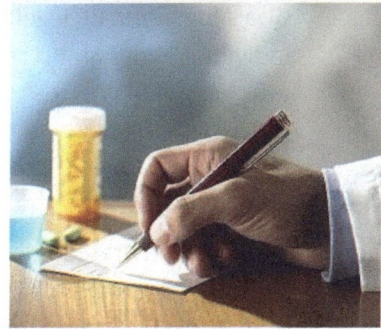

millionhearts.hhs.gov/tools-protocols/tools/cholesterol-management.html

The AHA has the following recommendations.[16]

- Statin therapy with intensive lipid-lowering effects (atorvastatin or rosuvastatin) is recommended to reduce the risk of stroke and cardiovascular events among patients with ischemic stroke or TIA presumed to be of atherosclerotic origin and an LDL (bad) cholesterol level ≥100 mg/dL with or without evidence for other ASCVD (atherosclerotic cardiovascular disease).

- Statin therapy with intensive lipid-lowering effects is recommended to reduce risk of the stroke and cardiovascular events among patients who have suffered an ischemic stroke or TIA presumed to be of atherosclerotic origin, an LDL cholesterol level <100 mg/dL and no evidence for other clinical ASCVD.

- Patients with ischemic stroke or TIA and other comorbid ASCVD should be otherwise managed according to the ACC/AHA 2013 guidelines, which include lifestyle modifications, dietary and medication recommendations.

Regarding blood pressure management, AHA recommends

---

[16] 2013 ACC/AHA Guideline on the Treatment of Blood Cholesterol to Reduce Atherosclerotic Cardiovascular Risk in Adults
Journal of the American College of Cardiology Volume 63, Issue 25 Part B, July 2014
A Report of the American College of Cardiology/American Heart Association Task Force on Practice Guidelines
Neil J Stone, Jennifer G Robinson, Alice H Lichtenstein, C Noel Bairey Merz, Conrad B Blum, Robert H Eckel, Anne C Goldberg, David Gordon, Daniel Levy, Donald M Lloyd-Jones, Patrick McBride, J Sanford Schwartz, Susan T Shero, Sidney C. Smith Jr., Karol Watson and Peter WF Wilson

the following:

- Initiation of BP therapy is indicated for previously untreated patients with ischemic stroke or TIA who, after the first several days, have an established BP ≥140 mm Hg systolic or ≥ 90 mm Hg diastolic. Initiation of therapy for patients with BP < 140 mm Hg systolic and < 90 mm Hg diastolic has uncertain benefits.

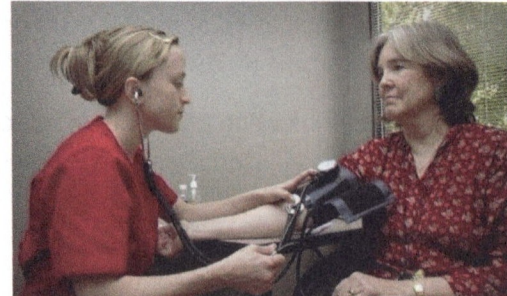

'Taking blood pressure'. Public Health Image Library. Public domain.

- Resumption of BP therapy is indicated for previously treated patients with known hypertension for both prevention of recurrent stroke and other vascular events in those who have had an ischemic stroke or TIA and are beyond the first several days.

- Goals for target BP level or reduction from pretreatment baseline are uncertain and should be individualized, but it is reasonable to achieve a systolic pressure < 140 mm Hg and a diastolic pressure < 90 mm Hg.

- For patients who suffered a lacunar stroke recently, it might be reasonable to target a systolic BP of < 130 mm Hg.

Research has demonstrated that most strokes are preventable. Everyone should be aware of how personal choices regarding tobacco use, diet and drug use have a tremendous impact on the risk of a disabling stroke. Furthermore, education on this matter evidently needs to focus on youth as well as adults of all ages. Patients with known risk factors should receive regular follow-up with healthcare providers who are knowledgeable about treatments for hypertension, hypercholesterolemia, diabetes and heart disease. Patients with prior stroke or TIA, atrial fibrillation or carotid stenosis should be considered for referral to specialists including neurologists, cardiologists, vascular surgeons or neurosurgeons.

You as an individual can assume an important role in educating Central Oregon about stroke risk factors and the importance of lifestyle choices and medical treatment. Just start by talking to your family and the message will spread from there.

Chapter 7. Stroke Outcomes and Overall Impact

St. Charles Medical System and Stroke Awareness Oregon have a mission to teach stroke awareness and to also reach out and support those recovering from stroke. We have a mission to teach hope. However, we must always be aware of the suffering and devastation created by the disease we are fighting.

One in every four people you know, including your closest family, is likely to suffer a stroke in their lifetime. We already learned in Chapter 1 that the lifetime stroke risk for Americans is 25%. Moreover, for patients who have suffered one stroke, there is a roughly 25% likelihood of a second stroke within five years.[17] There are over 795,000 new strokes that happen in the United States every year.[15] Two-thirds of stroke survivors are disabled.[15] The thought of stroke is often terrifying to people and many still believe that a stroke is the end of life. However, we know that through teaching stroke awareness and enabling people to access treatment early may save many people from death or devastating handicap. Unfortunately, we will never be able to prevent or treat all strokes. However, through rehabilitation, numerous survivors can regain independence and adapt to their impairments and thereby define quality of life in their terms.

---

[17] Heart disease and stroke statistics—2017 update: a report from the American Heart Association. Circulation. 2017;135:e229–e445.
Benjamin EJ, Blaha MJ, Chiuve SE, et al. on behalf of the American Heart Association Statistics Committee and Stroke Statistics Subcommittee.

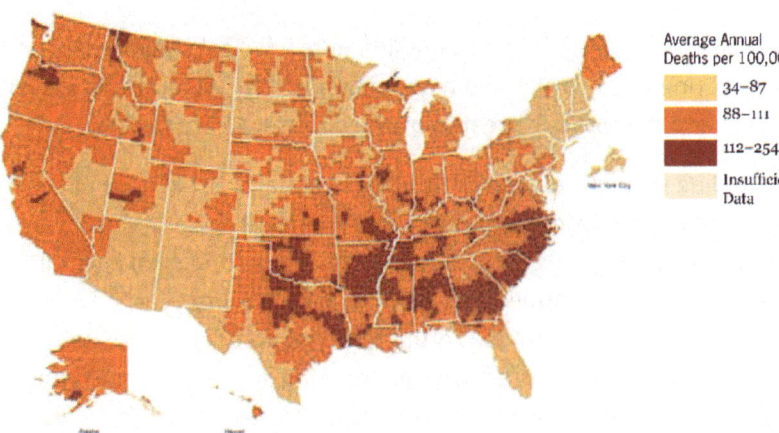

CDC / Public domain

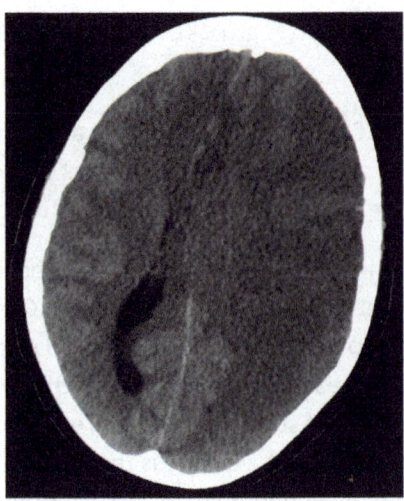

'Massive swelling from stroke resulting in midline shift and herniation'. James Heilman, MD / CC BY-SA
(https://creativecommons.org/licenses/by-sa/4.0)

Some strokes are so catastrophic that their outcome is death. The CDC reports that 140,000 people die each year from strokes.[18] Approximate 10–20% of strokes are fatal. People usually do not die immediately from stroke. At times, somebody will die immediately from a massive stroke, but more often, death is a result of complications that occur later, such as aspiration pneumonia, blood clots or infection. However, many severely affected stroke victims die from the sequence of brain injury itself as the ischemic brain tissue starts to swell. In an older brain, there's often enough brain atrophy (loss of brain tissue), thus there is space inside the skull to allow some swelling and brain expansion. Younger stroke victims do not have brain atrophy but may still suffer massive strokes in which brain swelling can compress other structures within the skull including arteries and veins. This leads to a spiral of further loss of blood flow, causing additional strokes and more swelling, eventually causing death. This process is known as brain **herniation** because the swollen brain will herniate through membrane compartments within the skull. Sometimes, hemorrhage within the stroke will hasten this process. Hemorrhage typically occurs within the first week and is seen more often in large strokes. The risk of **hemorrhagic conversion** of the stroke is one reason doctors sometimes have to temporarily postpone treatment with anticoagulant medications which are required to prevent additional strokes.

The loss of ability to swallow is a common feature in major strokes, particularly in older individuals who may have suffered previous strokes. This is known as **dysphagia**. All hospitalized patients who have strokes are carefully screened for dysphagia. Even then, stroke patients will often inhale any liquid or food in their mouth or their own saliva, leading to severe pneumonia. Thus, many patients with

---

[18] Vital Signs: Recent trends in stroke death rates – United States, 2000–2015. MMWR 2017;66.

dysphagia require nutrition either through a **nasogastric tube** or a permanent **gastrostomy**. Placement of the feeding tube requires permission of either the patient or family members who must make the decision based on their understanding of the patient's wishes.

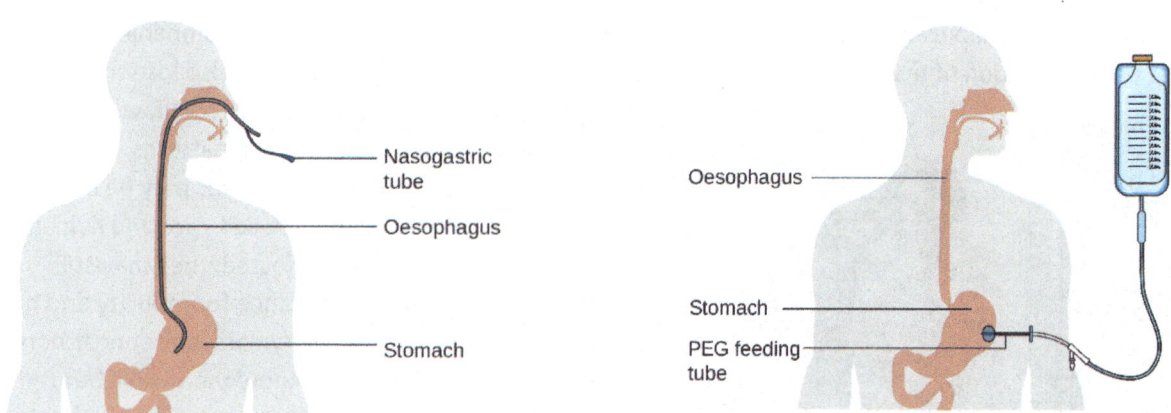

Cancer Research UK / CC BY-SA (https://creativecommons.org/licenses/by-sa/4.0)

Often, this is an extremely decision for families. Living wills, advance directives or a completed **POLST** form (Provider Orders for Life-Sustaining Treatment) becomes highly valuable in these usually unanticipated situations. Fortunately, for those who survive the initial stroke, most will recover enough swallowing ability so that swallowing therapy given by a speech therapist and changes in food consistencies can help avoid the need for a permanent feeding tube.

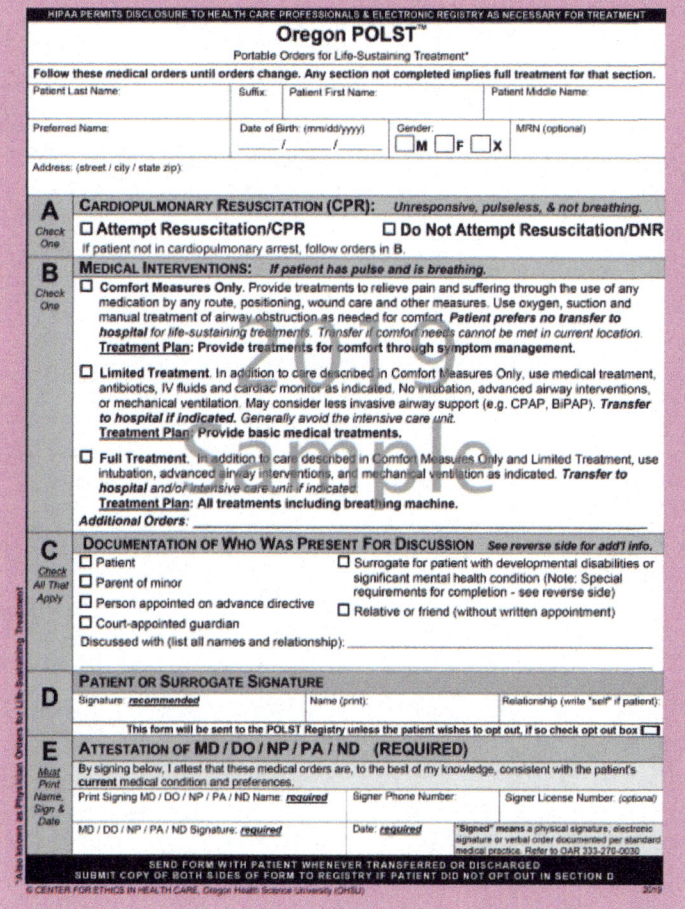

https://oregonpolst.org/

Stroke survivors may be left with varying degrees of disabilities ranging from mild to severe. Handicaps are extremely variable and often occur in combination. Limb weakness is usually accompanied by severe loss of coordination of the affected limb. Patients who have lost speech frequently also lose the ability to read or write and possibly swallow. Visual handicaps occur in multiple patterns. Survivors who have combined handicaps may be incapable of performing even basic self-care and hygiene. Even if less severely affected, they may still require constant assistance for mobility and basic needs. Some stroke survivors may appear normal to others who do not know them well, but the affected person may be struggling with impaired ability to make decisions or plan or understand what is happening around them. According to the American Stroke Association, 10% of people who experience a stroke recover almost completely, with 25% recovering with minor impairments. Another 40% experience moderate to severe impairments that require special care.

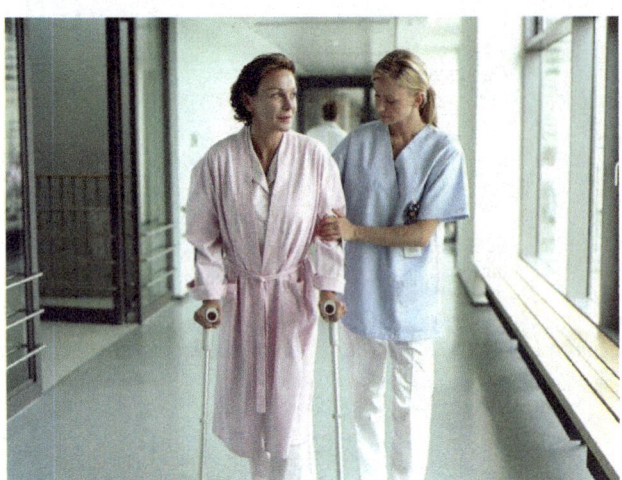
cdc.gov/stroke/recovery.htm

After the brain begins to heal from a stroke, sick brain cells may turn on again. Other dormant brain cells may be recruited to take over the function of cells that have died. Brain cells will sprout new connections and new brain pathways will develop. It is said that the brain is plastic. The process of brain rewiring is known as **plasticity**. There is tremendous plasticity in the children's brains, but this gradually declines as we age. Nonetheless, even elderly individuals can experience remarkable recovery after stroke. All of this stakes time though. Roughly, a person can expect to achieve 90% of their recovery by six months and 100% of the recovery within two years. But, if left alone, a stroke survivor who has not received therapy will never attain the remarkable recovery that is possible through intensive therapies.

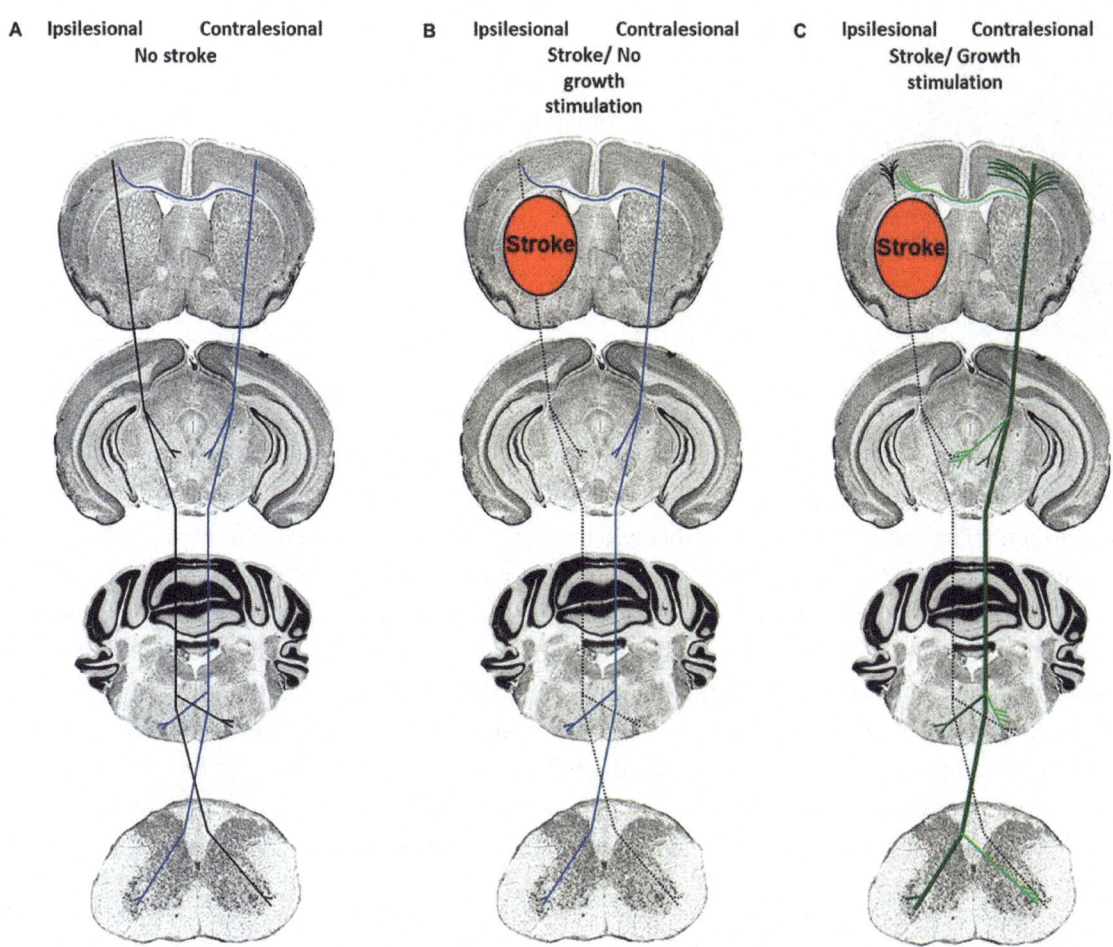

Neuronal plasticity features of cortical neurons in response to stroke and neuronal growth stimulation. Rat model. A. Normal pyramidal tracts. B. Atrophy of pyramidal tracts on left in response to stroke. C. After a period of recovery, abundant sprouting of pathways from the opposite cerebral hemisphere has occurred. Sanchez-Mendoza EH and Hermann DM (2016) Correlates of Post-Stroke Brain Plasticity, Relationship to Pathophysiological Settings and Implications for Human Proof-of-Concept Studies. Front. Cell. Neurosci. 10:196. doi: 10.3389/fncel.2016.00196. CC BY 4.0.

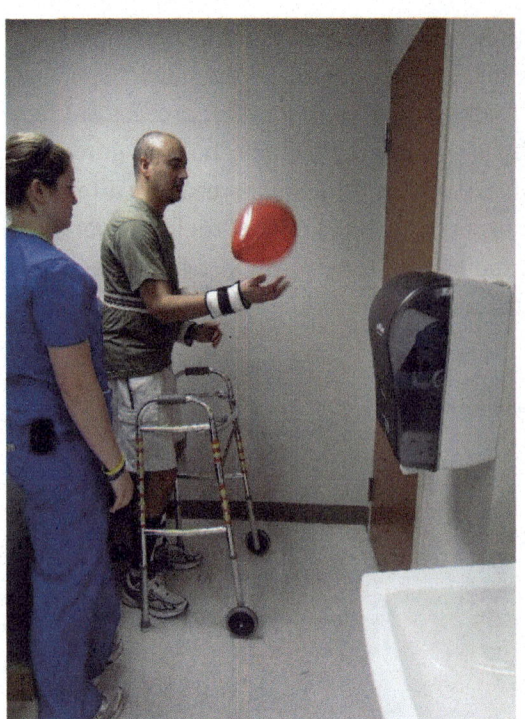

During initial hospitalization, stroke patients are seen by therapists as soon as they are medically stable enough to participate in therapies. Assessments by speech therapy for swallow safety and communication, mobility safety by physical therapy and the ability to perform basic care like dressing, toileting and bathing by occupational therapy are performed. For those with minimal impairments, this may be all the rehabilitation they require. However, most stroke patients need an extended rehabilitation program. **Physical medicine and rehabilitation specialists**, also known as "rehab doctors" or **physiatrists** should be consulted to identify which rehabilitation setting would be the most suitable for a patient for their recovery from residual impairments caused by stroke.

Roger Mommaerts / CC BY-SA
(https://creativecommons.org/licenses/by-sa/2.0)

About 22% patients were in an inpatient rehabilitation unit, 32% in a skilled nursing facility, 15% in a home health program, but 31% received no rehabilitation at all. The number of stroke survivors receiving no rehabilitation is climbing, possibly due to several factors. However, the high cost of care is likely a major cause. It is also important to remember that patients will often transition between these different types of rehabilitation programs as they improve. Some patients may use all of them. Many patients who can tolerate at least 3 hours of daily therapy and who are likely to eventually reenter the community may qualify for admission to the inpatient rehabilitation unit under the supervision of a rehab doctor. In the inpatient rehabilitation unit, concentrated multimodality therapy under supervision of different types of therapists greatly increases the possibility of good recovery and the very best possible outcome. However, all of this is highly regulated by Medicare which has strict rules for qualifying for these programs. Recovery is a journey. That journey can take 1–2 years to complete and often continues for years.

There are several methods of therapy that apply to stroke recovery. The subject is too extensive to cover in this concise review, but a few approaches will be discussed.

Task-specific training. This emphasizes repetitive practice of skilled motor performance to improve individuals' functional abilities necessary for daily living such as reaching, grasping, standing and

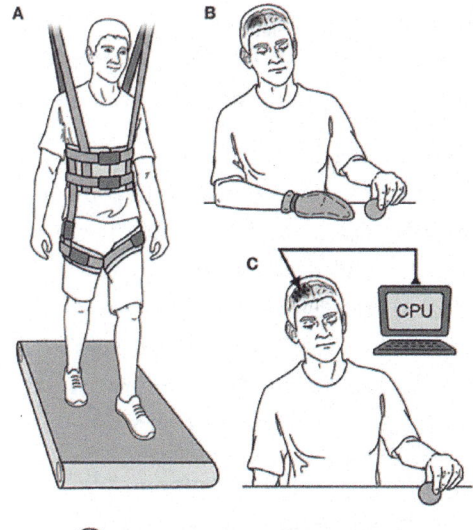

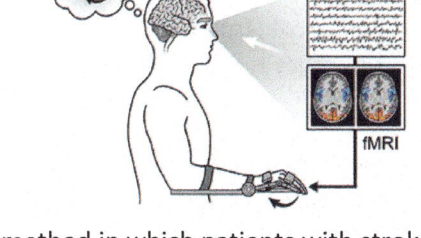

walking. Rather than simply attempting to exercise basic movements, directing the stroke patient to repeatedly perform specific complex tasks enhances adaptive neural plasticity.

Enriched environment. Therapy in a stroke unit or rehabilitation unit involves an organized package of care through a cyclical process. Patients learn what is expected of them during task-specific training. Patient involvement in interdisciplinary goal setting has shown to boost motivation and engagement as well as outcomes.

Novel approaches include CIMT (**constraint induced movement therapy**) in which the unaffected limb is physically restrained with a sling or glove. The repetitive training of the paralyzed limb may greatly enhance adaptive plasticity and recovery.

Krucoff MO, Rahimpour S, Slutzky MW, Edgerton VR and Turner DA (2016) Enhancing Nervous System Recovery through Neurobiologics, Neural Interface Training, and Neurorehabilitation. Front. Neurosci. 10:584. doi: 10.3389/fnins.2016.00584. CC BY 4.0

Moreover, BWSTT (**body weight support treadmill training**) is a method in which patients with stroke walk on a treadmill with their body weight partially supported. This enhances coverage of a normal gait and inhibits the development of abnormal walking patterns that often occur during stroke recovery.

Speech and language are the most important functions of the human brain. It concerns how we communicate information and ideas as well as our mood and feelings. These are necessary functions to live in society. **Aphasia**, loss of verbal comprehension and expressive language or speech is one of the most disabling features of stroke affecting the dominant left hemisphere.

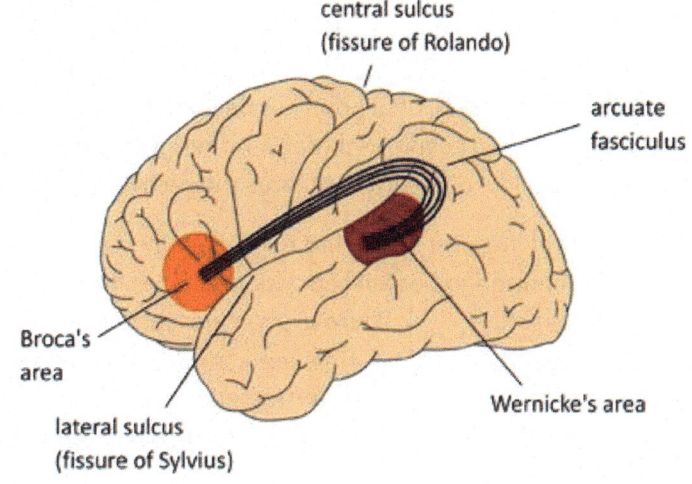

'In this model, Broca's area is crucial for language production, Wernicke's area subserves language comprehension, and the necessary information exchange between these areas (such as in reading aloud) is done via the arcuate fasciculus, a major fiber bundle connecting the language areas in the temporal cortex (Wernicke's area) and frontal cortex (Broca's area)'. By Peter Hagoort - Hagoort P (2013) MUC (Memory, Unification, Control) and beyond. Front. Psychol. 4:416. doi: 10.3389/fpsyg.2013., CC BY 3.0.

Aphasia can also affect reading and writing. The treatment of aphasia can focus on restorative approaches to improve or restore impaired language function of organs with compensatory approaches. Several strategies can be adopted to this end.

However, some stroke survivors suffer impairments so severe that 24-hour care is necessary. Quite frequently, this is something families are unable to provide. Huge barriers such as the need to provide care throughout the night as well as during the day or dealing with bowel or bladder incontinence are impossible for caregivers who need to work their regular job during the day. How well the stroke survivor can move and how much physical assistance required can also be a significant barrier to going home. The severely affected stroke victims may require transfer from the hospital to a **skilled nursing facility** to see if they can recover enough to return for inpatient rehabilitation or possibly return home. Some of these patients do not improve and eventually are transferred to an **extended care facility**.

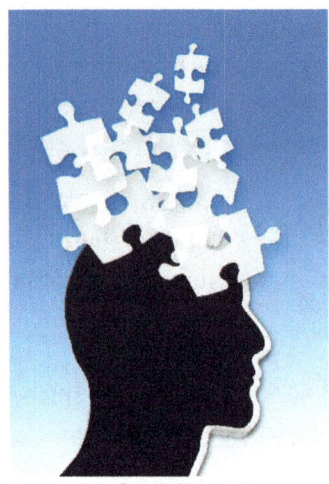
Image by Gerd Altmann. Pixabay

Handicaps from stroke are different from a broken leg or amputation because there is also an impact on a person's mind. Cognitive disability may be a part of their handicap. **Post-stroke cognitive impairment** or **post-stroke dementia** may affect up to one third of stroke survivors. Furthermore, stroke may hasten the onset of other types of dementia including Alzheimer's disease.

Many stroke survivors who do not suffer cognitive impairment still experience depression and loss of energy. Even a year later, half of stroke survivors identify loss of energy as their most troublesome symptom.

At least 25% of stroke survivors experience depression. This rate is considerably higher than that observed in patients who have suffered disabilities due to non-neurological causes. Some abnormal biological process occurs in stroke patients that lead to this significant problem.

Depression may be more common in patients who have experienced it before, but nobody is completely spared. Depression removes the joy of life and greatly hampers the recovery process. Many individuals with post stroke depression have no insight that they feel sad. Healthcare professionals and family members more often than not also fail to recognize the symptoms. However, post stroke depression is treatable. Coping strategies can be taught or encouraged. Antidepressant medications can be effective for mild to moderate depression. Often, medication is needed only temporarily. Additionally, counselors can help with a variety of approaches, including cognitive behavioral therapy, interpersonal therapy and mindfulness-based cognitive therapy. Adhering to a healthy lifestyle with good diet, exercise and avoidance of alcohol, clearly facilitates the recovery process as well.

The quality of life after stroke has been examined extensively. Overall, 52% to 82% of long-term stroke survivors reported to be satisfied with their lives. However, 23% reported low life satisfaction in one study. In that study, 30% of stroke survivors appear depressed according to test scores. Items that positively impacted quality-of-life perception was their relationship with family and the level of support in the community. Things that were rated important as negative factors in their perception of quality of life included inability to have a job, for individuals aged below 60. Reduced quality of sex life was also rated as important.

Furthermore, the financial impact of stroke care is tremendous. In 2014, nearly 8,000 people were hospitalized for stroke in Oregon, with an estimated cost of $146 million for hospital care.[19] While this is the cost of direct care, long-term follow-up entails additional costs, nursing home costs and indirect costs including loss of employability and income. The aggregate total cost total cost for stroke care exceeds $40 billion per year nationally.

One Billion Dollars. Roughly 1/40th of the yearly national cost of post-stroke care. Michael Marcovici / CC BY

Therefore, the impact of stroke on a person's life and community can be measured to some extent, and it is indeed massive. Nonetheless, people are born with incredible coping skills, and adaptability to life after stroke can be extremely good. Intensive rehabilitation, family support and community support are crucial in this. New treatments for stroke also manage to save a large number of people from devastating disabilities. However, none of this can continue if we leave the work to others. All of us, by teaching the message of FAST and sharing our knowledge with our families and community, must help in the process.

---

[19] The Oregon Stroke Care Committee Report to the 2017 Legislature

Made in the USA
Columbia, SC
01 February 2022